Review Questions for the **NCLEX–PN**

COMPUTERIZED ADAPTIVE TESTING

Third Edition

Review Questions for the

NCLEX–PN

Computerized Adaptive Testing

Third Edition

Sandra F. Smith, RN, MS

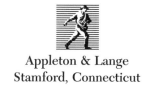

Appleton & Lange
Stamford, Connecticut

Copyright © 1997 by Appleton & Lange
A Simon & Schuster Company
Copyright © 1995, 1990 by National Nursing Review

97 98 99 00 01 / 10 9 8 7 6 5 4 3 2 1

Prentice Hall International (UK) Limited, *London*
Prentice Hall of Australia Pty. Limited, *Sydney*
Prentice Hall Canada, Inc., *Toronto*
Prentice Hall Hispanoamericana, S.A., *Mexico*
Prentice Hall of India Private Limited, *New Delhi*
Prentice Hall of Japan, Inc., *Tokyo*
Simon & Schuster Asia Pte. Ltd., *Singapore*
Editora Prentice Hall do Brasil Ltda., *Rio de Janeiro*
Prentice Hall, *Upper Saddle River, New Jersey*

Acquisitions Editor: David P. Carroll
Production Services: Forbes Mill Press
Cover Designer: Janice Barsevich Bielawa

PRINTED IN THE UNITED STATES OF AMERICA

ISBN 0-8385-8445-4

90000

9 780838 584453

Contents

Contributing Authors

Donna J. Duell, RN, MS, ABD
Cabrillo College
Aptos, California

Kyra Hubis, RN, MSN
Evergreen Valley College
San Jose, California

Marianne Hultgren, RN, MS
Cabrillo College
Aptos, California

Barbara Martin, RN, MS
University of Tulsa
Tulsa, Oklahoma

Sandra Fucci Smith, RN, MS, ABD
President, National Nursing Review
Los Altos, California

Russlyn A. St. John, RN, MSN
St. Charles County Community College
St. Peters, Missouri

Dolores Vaz, RN, MSN, MEd
Bristol Community College
Fall River, Massachusetts

Preface

The purpose of the National Council Licensure Examination (NCLEX) is to ensure that candidates for PN licensure are qualified to practice safe, effective entry-level nursing care. Passing the NCLEX is an important milestone in your nursing career. ***Review Questions for the NCLEX-PN CAT*** was written to assist you to prepare for and pass this examination.

In addition to containing challenging simulated NCLEX test questions, this book provides the licensure candidate with important information about the NCLEX-PN and how to prepare for it. The National Council's Test Plan is described and illustrated with sample questions. Review guidelines and test-taking strategies are presented to help you plan your review time efficiently and to become comfortable with the format and style of NCLEX questions. Special attention is devoted to explaining Computerized Adaptive Testing and computer testing tips. You can rehearse taking the NCLEX by using the computer disk that accompanies this book. With a greater understanding of the purpose of the test and its associated procedures, you should feel more confident concerning how to prepare for it.

The comprehensive tests and individual subject/clinical area questions serve two purposes: (1) to acquaint you with the type of questions to expect on the examination, and (2) to give you an opportunity to test and improve your knowledge of nurse-client clinical situations. The answers-and-rationale sections are intended to discourage rote memorization and to reinforce learning by describing the underlying principles that explain why the answers are right or wrong. The selection of the content in this book is directed toward minimizing your review time and maximizing your test results.

Review Questions for the NCLEX-PN CAT is dedicated to the many nursing students who, after several years of classroom study and clinical experience, face the crucial examination for PN licensure. If this text and the accompanying computer disk help you prepare more fully and enter your test session with increased confidence, the project will be considered an unqualified success by the author.

Acknowledgments

I wish to extend my thanks to all of the contributing authors and to many others who helped with the development of this book. Because of their valuable assistance, this book is available to help candidates prepare for the current PN licensure examination.

Sandra F. Smith

I

PREPARING FOR THE NCLEX-PN CAT

PN/VN Licensure Procedures

The Purpose of NCLEX

The National Council Licensure Examination for Practical Nurses (commonly abbreviated to NCLEX-PN*) measures the licensure candidate's competence to perform safe and effective entry-level nursing practice. The boards of nursing in all 50 states, the District of Columbia, and the U.S. territories of Guam, the Virgin Islands, American Samoa, Puerto Rico, and the Northern Mariana Islands administer this screening test as developed by the National Council of State Boards of Nursing (NCSBN). This system of licensure provides protection for health care consumers and defines common entry-level standards throughout the U.S. In order to take the NCLEX, the candidate for licensure applies to the board of nursing in the state or jurisdiction in which the candidate plans to practice nursing. A complete list of the State Boards of Nursing is included as Appendix 2.

The NCLEX-PN Test Plan Framework

The National Council is responsible to provide its member boards of nursing with a psychometrically sound and legally defensible licensure examination. The purpose of the NCLEX-PN is to separate licensure candidates into two groups: those who can demonstrate minimal competence to perform safe and effective entry-level nursing care, and those who cannot.

Administration of the test via Computerized Adaptive Testing (CAT) was implemented in 1994. The current test plan that provides the framework for presenting the questions became effective in October 1996. The National Council contracts with clinical nurses and nurse educators to write questions (referred to as test items) that test your ability to apply your knowledge of vocational/practical nursing. The test questions focus on job tasks normally performed by entry-level PNs during their first 6 to 12 months on the job. The National Council identifies these tasks by conducting extensive surveys, called job analysis studies, about every three years.

It is very possible that your PN program may have included instruction on certain tasks that are not considered to be entry level by the National Council's job analysis study. It is also possible that your PN program may not have provided you with instruction on some of the tasks about which questions have been included in the current test pool.

---

* NCLEX-PN is a registered trademark of the National Council of State Boards of Nursing, Inc.

The job analysis studies are also used to help validate the test plan and to provide the basis for the proportional distribution of questions among the various subjects covered by the test. The test's two most significant conceptual areas are the Nursing Process and Client Needs. The following sections describe each phase of the Nursing Process, define the four broad categories of Client Needs, and list the 11 subcategories of Client Needs.

The Nursing Process

The phases of the Nursing Process that are measured by the NCLEX-PN include Data Collection, Planning, Implementation, and Evaluation. The accompanying chart shows the percentage of questions that are allocated to each phase.

Nursing Process	Question Allocation
Data Collection	27–33%
Planning	17–23%
Implementation	27–33%
Evaluation	17–29%

By definition, *process* is a series of actions that leads toward a particular result. When attached to *nursing*, the term *Nursing Process* becomes a general description of a nurse's job: collecting data, planning, implementing, and evaluating. The objective of this process of decision-making is to promote optimal health care for clients. While the steps can be described separately and in logical order, it is obvious that in practice the steps will overlap. Events may not always occur in the order listed above, especially when the unexpected happens. However, for purposes of understanding the NCLEX test plan, it is appropriate to work through each phase in a logical progression.

Data Collection

The data collection phase refers to building a data base for a specific client. This phase requires skilled observation and collection of data from the client, family, health team members, and medical records. It also includes a theoretical knowledge base to gather and differentiate data and to document findings. The practical nurse gathers information relevant to the patient, assigns meaning to this data, and uses it to participate in the formulation of a nursing diagnosis. For example:

> A 1-year-old child, with severe diarrhea of 2 days duration, is admitted to a hospital. His temperature is 37.8°C (100°F). Upon admission, the most important assessment is to
>
> 1. Determine the child's weight.
> 2. Take the child's apical-radial pulse.
> 3. Check the child's respirations.
> 4. Check the child's skin turgor.

The answer is (4). The most important nursing observation is to check the child's hydration status, and this can be determined by assessing skin turgor. This is the most critical assessment, as small children have so little body surface that they can die from severe dehydration.

Planning

Based on data collected, the planning phase refers to identifying goals of care. The practical nurse contributes to the nursing care plan, assists in formulating goals, and communicates client needs and nursing measures necessary to achieve goals. This phase of the nursing process also includes nursing measures for the delivery of care. Clients may be involved in this planning phase. A planning question will focus on the development of a plan of care individualized for a specific client.

A depressed client becomes more active and her mood has lifted. An appropriate goal to add to the nursing care plan is to
1. Encourage the client to go home for the weekend.
2. Move the client to a room with three other clients.
3. Monitor the client's whereabouts at all times.
4. Begin to explore the reasons the client became depressed.

The answer is (3). The goal is to implement suicide precautions because the danger of suicide occurs when the depression lifts and the client has the energy to formulate a plan.

Implementation

The third phase of the nursing process is the implementation or intervention phase. This phase refers to the interventions performed to accomplish specified goals. It describes the action component of the nursing process. This phase involves initiating and completing the nursing actions necessary to accomplish the identified client goals. Implementation includes performing basic therapeutic and preventive nursing measures, providing a safe and effective environment, recording and reporting specific information, and assisting the client to understand the care plan.

Implementation of the plan involves giving direct care to the client to accomplish the specified goal.

The nurse's assessment of a client indicates evidence of increasing intracranial pressure. The first nursing action is to
1. Attempt to have the client take slow, deep breaths.
2. Place the client in high-Fowler's position.
3. Place the client on his side.
4. Have the client cough and deep breathe.

The answer is (1). As the $PaCO_2$ increases in the cerebral tissues, blood rushes to the area and this further increases the intracranial pressure. Decreasing the $PaCO_2$, accomplished by breathing deeper and more slowly, will increase the intracranial blood flow, thus decreasing intracranial pressure.

Evaluation

The final phase of the nursing process is evaluation, or determining the extent to which the plan or identified goals were achieved. Evaluation is the examination of the client's response or the outcome of nursing interventions. This process is extremely important, because without this step, the nursing plan cannot be evaluated and adapted to the client's ongoing needs.

The nurse will know that a client with gouty arthritis needs more teaching about his diet when he says he can eat
1. As much fish and chicken as he wishes.
2. Fresh vegetables and eggs every day.
3. At least 2 fruits per day.
4. No organ meats.

The answer is (1). A client with gout must avoid foods high in purine (meats, fish and legumes are relatively high in purine). Fresh vegetables, fruits and eggs are low in purine.

Client Needs

The basic health needs of clients are grouped under four broad categories that are weighted according to the results of a job analysis study completed in 1994. The weight assigned to each category is reflected in the percentage of questions you will find on the current NCLEX as noted in the accompanying chart.

Client Needs	Question Allocation
Safe, Effective Care Environment	16–22%
Physiological Integrity	49–55%
Psychosocial Integrity	8–14%
Health Promotion and Maintenance	15–21%

Safe, Effective Care Environment

To assist in meeting the client's needs in this area, the practical nurse must be able to provide the following:

- Coordinated Care
- Environmental Safety
- Safe and Effective Treatments and Procedures †

Physiological Integrity

To assist in meeting the client's needs for physiological integrity—this includes acute and/or chronically recurring physiological conditions, as well as potential complications—the practical nurse must be able to provide nursing care in the following areas:

- Physiological Adaptation
- Reduction of Risk Potential †
- Provision of Basic Care †

Psychosocial Integrity

To assist in meeting the client's needs for psychosocial integrity during periods of illness and common health problems that occur throughout the life cycle, the practical nurse must be able to provide nursing care in the following areas:

- Psychosocial Adaptation
- Coping/Adaptation †

Health Promotion and Maintenance

To assist in meeting the client's needs for health promotion and maintenance throughout the life cycle, the practical nurse must be able to provide nursing care in the following areas:

- Continued Growth and Development Through the Life Span
- Self-Care and Support Systems †
- Prevention and Early Treatment of Disease

---

† Indicates areas of greater job importance; therefore, more emphasis is given to presenting questions in these subcategories.

Adapted from **NCLEX-PN Test Plan for the National Council Licensure Examination for Practical Nurses**, National Council of State Boards of Nursing, Chicago, 1995.

Computerized Adaptive Testing

CAT Background

With the introduction of Computerized Adaptive Testing (CAT) in 1994, the procedures for taking the NCLEX changed radically from prior protocol. The major new elements include:

1. Locating test sites throughout the U.S. where each candidate makes an appointment to take the test on an individual basis.

2. Presenting the test on a computer screen rather than in a printed test booklet. Answer selections are made by pressing keys on a computer keyboard instead of marking an answer sheet with a pencil.

3. Generating a unique test for each candidate because the computer selects each subsequent question based upon the candidate's prior answers.

The Advantages of CAT

CAT is described as providing a more comfortable and convenient way to take NCLEX. The testing environment at a Sylvan Technology Center will be similar to a small classroom or learning laboratory, in contrast to a large hall or convention center with the distractions and tension associated with a large group of candidates taking the test simultaneously. From a procedural standpoint, the advantages of CAT are defined as:

1. A more efficient way to test and measure competency than the prior pencil and paper test format.

2. Reduction of testing time to a maximum of five hours in one test session.

3. Greater security and the avoidance of inconvenience to candidates if security measures break down.

4. Year-round testing schedules that provide applicants with greater flexibility and convenience than the prior twice-per-year system.

5. Substantial reduction in the time required between applying to take NCLEX and receiving one's results.

Administrative Organizations

Three organizations are involved with administering NCLEX: (1) Boards of Nursing from each state or jurisdiction, (2) the Educational Testing Service (ETS), and (3) Sylvan Learning Systems. As a candidate for licensure, it will help you to know the role of each organization.

As described earlier in this section, the National Council designs the test plan, conducts the job analysis, and sets the passing standard. Educational Testing Service formulates the test questions to conform to the National Council's Test Plan. ETS maintains a test pool of several thousand questions written by specially selected item writers approved by the state boards of nursing. All NCLEX questions are drawn from this test pool. You will make an appointment with and physically take the NCLEX-PN at a Sylvan Technology Center. Approximately 200 of these centers are available throughout the U.S. for NCLEX testing.

Application Procedures

After the state (jurisdiction) in which you plan to practice accepts your application and verifies your eligibility to take the NCLEX, you will receive an Authorization to Test and other information that includes the locations and telephone numbers of the Sylvan Technology Centers. You will then contact a test center of your choice to make an appointment to take the test. The test center does not need to be located in the state to which you have applied for licensure. As a first time test taker, you should be able to schedule your appointment within 30 days of your call. Read all instructions carefully, especially noting the items that you must bring to the test center.

Taking the NCLEX

Upon arriving at the Sylvan Technology Center, you will present your Authorization to Test and two forms of identification, both signed and one with a photo. A driver's license, school or employee I.D., and passport are the most accepted forms. A social security card is an example of an unacceptable proof of identity. At check-in, you will be photographed and thumbprinted.

Before commencing the test questions, you will complete a brief computer tutorial to make certain that you are comfortable with the keyboard procedures. The National Council advises that no prior computer experience is necessary for CAT.

Two types of questions appear on NCLEX. The *real* questions test your competency and safety and provide the basis for your pass or fail score. The *tryout* questions are items being field tested for future NCLEX exams. You have no way of knowing the difference between real and tryout.

The minimum number of questions for each candidate will be 60 real and 15 to 25 tryout for a total of 75 to 85. The National Council maintains that the essential Test Plan categories can be covered by 60 carefully selected questions. The maximum number of real questions is 180, so by adding the 15 to 25 tryouts, you could answer a total of 205 items.

CAT does not allow you to skip questions, change answers, or go back to look at questions already answered. Each question has an assigned degree of difficulty. Based on your prior answers—correct or incorrect—the computer selects the next question. Therefore, you must answer each question as it is presented. Because the computer draws from a large pool of questions, each candidate's test is unique. There is no absolute passing score in terms of the number or percent of questions that you must answer correctly in order to pass.

After you have answered the minimum number of questions, your test continues until the computer calculates with a 95% degree of confidence that you fall into the safe/competent group or that you do not. Although there is no minimum amount of time for your test, the maximum allowable test duration is five hours, including your computer tutorial and rest breaks. A mandatory rest break of 10 minutes is required after two hours of testing and an optional break is available after the next one and one-half hours.

Getting Your Test Results

The results of your test are electronically transmitted from the Sylvan Technology Center where you take the test to Educational Testing Service in Princeton, New Jersey, for processing. Within 48 hours, ETS forwards your results to the board of nursing to which you applied for licensure. Your results—pass or fail—will be sent to you by the board of nursing. The time required for the board of nursing to notify the candidate will vary from state to state.

An NCLEX Candidate Diagnostic Profile is provided for all failure candidates. There are three types of diagnostic profile reports. The majority of candidates receive a diagnostic profile like the one shown in Appendix 1. This profile includes identifying candidate information, describes the candidate's overall performance on the examination and the number of items answered, and provides information on the candidate's performance in each area of the Phases of the Nursing Process and the Categories of Client Needs to assist the candidate to study for the next examination. The reverse side of the NCLEX Candidate Diagnostic Profile contains the test plan definitions.

Slightly different information is presented in the diagnostic profile for candidates who have not demonstrated competency before their time expires. These candidates do not receive an overall performance assessment.

Candidates who do not complete at least the minimum number of items receive a report which states that a diagnostic report cannot be provided. Insufficient information is available to provide a diagnostic report.

NCLEX Information on the Web

An interactive version of the NCLEX Diagnostic Profile can be accessed on the National Council's World Wide Web site at http://www.ncsbn.org. The objective of this interactive program is to help the candidate interpret the information contained on her/his diagnostic profile and to provide guidance for follow-up review and study. Other material accessible on the National Council's Web site includes (a) overview of the NCLEX testing process, (b) registering for the test and scheduling an appointment, (c) description of Computerized Adaptive Testing, and (d) NCLEX passing rates.

NCLEX-PN CAT Quick Reference
Test Location: Sylvan Technology Centers
Minimum Number of Questions: 75 to 85
Maximum Number of Questions: 195 to 205
Minimum Testing Time: None
Maximum Testing Time: 5 hours

Appendix 1. NCLEX-PN™ Candidate Diagnostic Profile
National Council Licensure Examination for Practical Nurses

NATIONAL COUNCIL National Council of State Boards of Nursing, Inc.

Test Date: 10/25/96
Test Center: 51807

Candidate Number: 800-75-970
Date of Birth: 01/16/75
Social Security Number: 546-46-8861
Program Code: 49-198
Program Name: Southeastern Illinois Coll
A   Harrisburg, IL
    Brenda Jones
    PO Box 15
    Harrisburg, IL 61234

Candidate's Photograph Here

Brenda Jones, an applicant for licensure by the
ILLINOIS DEPT. OF PROFESSIONAL REGULATION,
HAS NOT PASSED the National Council Licensure Examination

The scale below, titled "Overall Performance Assessment," show how well you did on the NCLEX-PN. The "X" shows how far below passing your performance fell. Passing is indicated by the "|" shown in the box.

On the NCLEX-PN, no candidate is administered more than 205 questions. The box title "Number of Items Taken" shows that the computer reached a decision after you had answered   205   questions.

"Only candidates whose performance was close to the passing standard, either just above or just below it, had to answer the maximum number of 205 questions. For candidates whose performance was much higher or much lower than the passing standard, fewer questions were required before a confident pass or fail decision could be made."

The back of this form lists the eight test plan content areas. The "X" in the eight boxes at the bottom of this page show how well you did in those content areas. This will help you know which areas to study before you take the test again.

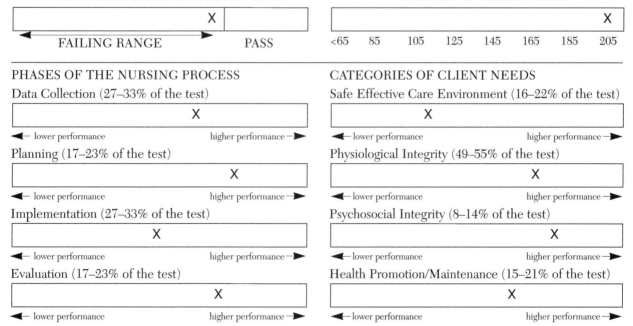

OVERALL PERFORMANCE ASSESSMENT

| | X | |

← FAILING RANGE → PASS

NUMBER OF ITEMS TAKEN

| | X |

<65   85   105   125   145   165   185   205

PHASES OF THE NURSING PROCESS
Data Collection (27–33% of the test)

| X |

◄— lower performance   higher performance —►

Planning (17–23% of the test)

| X |

◄— lower performance   higher performance —►

Implementation (27–33% of the test)

| X |

◄— lower performance   higher performance —►

Evaluation (17–23% of the test)

| X |

◄— lower performance   higher performance —►

CATEGORIES OF CLIENT NEEDS
Safe Effective Care Environment (16–22% of the test)

| X |

◄— lower performance   higher performance —►

Physiological Integrity (49–55% of the test)

| X |

◄— lower performance   higher performance —►

Psychosocial Integrity (8–14% of the test)

| X |

◄— lower performance   higher performance —►

Health Promotion/Maintenance (15–21% of the test)

| X |

◄— lower performance   higher performance —►

Printed by permission of the National Council of State Boards of Nursing, Inc., Chicago, IL

Appendix 2. Directory of Boards of Nursing

Executive Officer
Board of Nursing
P.O. Box 303900
Montgomery, Alabama 36130

Executive Secretary
Alaska Board of Nursing
3601 C Street, Suite 722
Anchorage, Alaska 99503

Secretary
Health Services Regulatory Board
LBJ Tropical Medical Center
Pago Pago, American Samoa 96799

Executive Director
Arizona State Board of Nursing
1651 E. Morton, Suite 150
Phoenix, Arizona 85020

Executive Director
Arkansas State Board of Nursing
1123 South University, Suite 800
Little Rock, Arkansas 72204

Executive Officer
Board of Vocational Nursing and
Psychiatric Technical Examiners
2535 Capitol Oaks Drive, Suite 205
Sacramento, California 95833

Program Administrator
Colorado State Board of Nursing
1560 Broadway, Suite 670
Denver, Colorado 80202

Executive Officer
Department of Health Services
410 Capitol Avenue MS 12 Nur.
P.O. Box 340308
Hartford, Connecticut 06134

Executive Director
Delaware Board of Nursing
P. O. Box 1401
Canon Building, Suite 203
Dover, Delaware 19903

Chairperson
District of Columbia Board of Nursing
614 H Street NW
Washington, DC 20013

Executive Director
Florida State Board of Nursing
111 E. Coastline Drive
Jacksonville, Florida 32202

Executive Director
Georgia Board of Examiners of
Licensed Practical Nurses
166 Pryor Street NW, Suite 300
Atlanta, Georgia 30303

Administrator
Guam Board of Nurse Examiners
P. O. Box 2816
Agana, Guam 96910

Executive Secretary
Hawaii Board of Nursing
Box 3469
Honolulu, Hawaii 99503

Executive Director
Idaho State Board of Nursing
P.O. Box 83720
Boise, Idaho 83720

Nursing Education Coordinator
Department of Professional Regulation
320 W. Washington Street
Springfield, Illinois 62786

Board Administration
Indiana State Board of Nursing
402 W. Washington Street
Indianapolis, Indiana 46204

Executive Director
Iowa Board of Nursing
1223 E. Court Avenue
Des Moines, Iowa 50319

Executive Administrator
Kansas State Board of Nursing
900 SW Jackson Street, Suite 551S
Topeka, Kansas 66612

Executive Director
Kentucky Board of Nursing
312 Whittington Pkwy, Suite 300
Louisville, Kentucky 40222

Executive Director
Louisiana State Board of PN Examiners
1440 Canal Street, Suite 1722
New Orleans, Louisiana 70112

Executive Director
Maine State Board of Nursing
35 Anthony Avenue
State House Station 158
Augusta, Maine 04333

Executive Director
Maryland Board of Nursing
4140 Patterson Avenue
Baltimore, Maryland 21215

Executive Secretary
Board of Registration in Nursing
100 Cambridge Street, Room 150
Boston, Massachusetts 02202

Board Secretary
Michigan Board of Nursing
P. O. Box 30018, 611 West Ottawa
Lansing, Michigan 48909

Executive Director
Minnesota Board of Nursing
2700 University Avenue, West 108
St. Paul, Minnesota 55114

Supervisor
Health Occupations Education
Division of Vocational Education
Department of Education
P. O. Box 771
Jackson, Mississippi 39205

Executive Director
Missouri State Board of Nursing
3605 Missouri Boulevard
Jefferson City, Missouri 65102

Executive Director
Montana State Board of Nursing
111 Jackson, Arcade Building
Helena, Montana 59620

Associate Director
Bureau of Examining Board
P. O. Box 95007
Lincoln, Nebraska 68509

Executive Director
Nevada State Board of Nursing
4335 S. Industrial Road, Suite 420
Las Vegas, Nevada 89103

Executive Director
State Board of Nursing
Division of Public Health
6 Hazen Drive
Concord, New Hampshire 03301

Executive Director
New Jersey Board of Nursing
P. O. Box 45010
Newark, New Jersey 07101

Executive Director
New Mexico Board of Nursing
4206 Louisiana NE, Suite A
Albuquerque, New Mexico 87109

Executive Secretary
New York State Board of Nursing
The Cultural Center, Room 3023
Albany, New York 12230

Executive Director
North Carolina Board of Nursing
P. O. Box 2129
Raleigh, North Carolina 27602

Executive Director
North Dakota Board of Nursing
919 S. 7th Street, Suite 504
Bismarck, North Dakota 58504

Executive Director
Ohio Board of Nursing
77 S. High Street, 17th Floor
Columbus, Ohio 43266

Executive Director
Oklahoma Board of Nursing
2915 N. Classen Boulevard, Suite 524
Oklahoma City, Oklahoma 73106

Executive Director
Oregon State Board of Nursing
800 NE Oregon Street, #25
Portland, Oregon 97232

Executive Secretary
Pennsylvania State Board of
Nurse Examiners
P. O. Box 2649
Harrisburg, Pennsylvania 17105

Director
Licensure Office
General Council on Education
P.O. Box 195429
San Juan, Puerto Rico 00910

Director
Board of Registration in Nursing
3 Capitol Hill
Providence, Rhode Island 02908

Executive Director
State Board of Nursing for
South Carolina
220 Executive Center Drive, Suite 220
Columbia, South Carolina 29210

Executive Secretary
South Dakota Board of Nursing
3307 South Lincoln
Sioux Falls, South Dakota 57105

Executive Director
Tennessee Board of Nursing
283 Plus Park Boulevard
Nashville, Tennessee 37217

Executive Director
Board of Vocational Nurse Examiners
9101 Burnet Road, Suite 105
Austin, Texas 78758

Executive Secretary
Utah State Board of Nursing
160 East 300 South, Box 45805
Salt Lake City, Utah 84145

Executive Director
Vermont Board of Nursing
Licensing and Registration Division
109 State Street
Montpelier, Vermont 05602

Executive Secretary
Virgin Islands Board of Nurse Licensure
P. O. Box 4247
Charlotte Amalie, Virgin Islands 00803

Executive Director
Virginia State Board of Nursing
6606 W. Broad Street, 4th Floor
Richmond, Virginia 23230

Executive Director
State Board of Practical Nursing
1300 Quince Street, P.O. Box 47864
Olympia, Washington 98504

Executive Secretary
Board of Examiners for Practical Nurses
101 Dee Drive
Charleston, West Virginia 25311

Administrative Officer
Wisconsin Department of Regulation &
Licensing
P. O. Box 8935
Madison, Wisconsin 53708

Executive Director
State of Wyoming Board of Nursing
2301 Central Avenue, Barrett Building
Cheyenne, Wyoming 82002

II

GUIDELINES FOR EFFECTIVE REVIEW AND TEST TAKING

Reviewing and Testing

Test Anxiety

A common source of test anxiety is the fear of not being sufficiently prepared to pass the test. This is very common among PN licensure candidates for a variety of reasons including:

1. Limited time available for review between the completion of final examinations and your appointment to take the NCLEX-PN.
2. Difficulty in motivation to begin concentrated study following the emotional and physical drain of finishing nursing school.
3. Inability to sort out and organize vast quantities of material to which you have been exposed during nursing school.
4. Absence of a defined study plan that includes a systematic review.
5. Lack of self-knowledge of your own strengths and weaknesses in terms of categories or subjects tested by the NCLEX-PN.
6. Uncertainty regarding the NCLEX-PN test plan, subject emphasis, or scoring procedures.
7. Lack of confidence that nursing school instruction effectively prepared you for the licensure examination.

There are many other reasons why candidates feel less than totally confident regarding NCLEX-PN, but the above list summarizes the major sources of test anxiety. Of course, when the candidate has high test anxiety, he or she may have difficulty even getting started on an effective review program.

Your Review Program

You want your review program to be effective and efficient. By effective, we mean that the program works—you enter the test site with calmness and confidence, and you pass. By efficient, we refer to the relationship between the results and the cost in time and money to achieve them.

The following recommendations illustrate ways that you can achieve maximum results for the amount of time invested.

1. Plan your study and review periods at regular intervals for best efficiency.
   a. Arrange to study when mentally alert; if you study during periods of mental and physical fatigue, your efficiency is reduced.
   b. When studying, use short breaks at relatively frequent intervals. Breaks used as rewards for hard work serve as incentives for continued concentrated effort.

2. Identify your strengths and weaknesses to enable you to efficiently focus your review time.

    a. Consider your past performance on classroom tests and written clinical applications of factual material. Learn from past errors on tests by studying corrected material.

    b. Use the Self-Assessment and Evaluation Grids contained in this book to help you identify your areas of strength and weakness.

    c. Systematically eliminate your weaknesses. Allow sufficient time for repeated review of those areas that continue to pose problems.

3. Familiarize yourself with the examination format and multiple choice tests.

    a. Study the format used for NCLEX-PN so that you will know the different ways in which questions are asked. For example, you must know how to deal with clinical situations and multiple-choice questions.

    b. Practice answering the questions in this book. Become familiar with how NCLEX questions are worded. Read the rationales that accompany the answers and build your body of knowledge.

4. Apply time management to taking multiple-choice tests.

    a. The total time allotment for you to complete your NCLEX CAT is 5 hours. However, it is still important that you practice time management with test questions, so that you are programmed not to spend too much time on any one question.

    b. You can prepare yourself to accomplish this by allotting 1 minute per question as you take practice tests. At the rate of 1 minute per question, you will be able to answer 205 questions in just under 3½ hours. This allows you the additional time to complete your computer tutorial and to take your required break. However, the NCLEX CAT appears to be designed to measure your competency in substantially fewer than the maximum of 205 questions.

5. Systematically study the material contained in a review book. You will find a complete review of nursing in **Content Review for the NCLEX-PN**, also by Sandra Smith.

    a. First gain a general impression of the chapter, or content unit, to be reviewed. Skim over the entire section. Observe how the material is organized and identify the main ideas.

    b. Systematically read through the material and, as appropriate, relate the content to the nursing process. Visualize the situations from a nurse-client decision making basis.

    c. Carefully read and study the tables and appendices where much factual background data is summarized. Using these quick reference sources will reduce time-consuming searches of textbooks or personal notes.

    d. Mark important material and note subjects that you do not know thoroughly for additional review.

6. Follow up on your priority areas.

    a. Set priorities on the material that is to be learned or reviewed. Identify the most crucial sections and underline the essential thoughts.

    b. Review what you have read. Ask yourself to think of examples that illustrate the main points you have studied. Recall examples from your own clinical experience or from clinical cases about which you have read.

     c.   Solidify newly learned material by writing down the main ideas or by explaining the major points to another person.

7.   Test yourself on what you have learned.

     a.   Answer the practice questions in this review book. Fill out the Self-Assessment Grids and check your progress.

     b.   Study the answers and their rationale. Concentrate on understanding the underlying principles and reasons for the answers.

     c.   Acquire the flexibility to answer questions phrased in different ways over the same wide range of content. Important concepts may be tested repeatedly in exams, but the questions will be worded differently.

     d.   Use the disk attached to the inside back cover of this book so that you become familiar with the computer screen format and the keyboard procedures for answering questions. Your Performance Summary will provide you with helpful feedback. Study the rationales for questions missed to understand why you answered those questions incorrectly.

Test-Taking Strategies for NCLEX

Understanding Test Construction

NCLEX-PN candidates who understand test construction and who utilize effective test-taking strategies generally perform better than candidates with a similar knowledge base who approach an examination without adequate skills in test-taking techniques. Fear of the unknown can contribute to pretest anxiety, and confusion at the test site can increase this anxiety. This section identifies and describes test-taking guidelines that have proven to be very helpful to candidates for PN licensure.

First, it is important to realize that a multiple choice test is very different from other types of tests such as essay, matching, and true/false. In multiple choice exams, the question is called the **stem**. The stem is followed by four alternative answers. One answer is correct, and the other three are referred to as **distractors** because they distract your attention from identifying and selecting the correct answer. It is important to understand that the distractors are not necessarily wrong, but rather they may not be **as** correct or **as** complete as the right answer.

The multiple choice questions in this book are similar in format, subject matter, length, and degree of difficulty to those contained in the NCLEX-PN. The answers to the multiple-choice questions are accompanied by rationale or an identification of the underlying principle. The answer sections provide you with an added learning experience; if you understand the basic principles of nursing content, you can transfer these principles to the clinical situations contained in the NCLEX-PN. Furthermore, the comprehensive tests will provide a basis for understanding the process of selecting the "best" answer to a question.

The following strategies will help you become better prepared to deal with various question types and to more efficiently compare and evaluate the answer selections.

Ten Useful Strategies

Strategy #1 Understand exactly what the stem is asking before considering the distractors.

Make sure you read the stem correctly. Notice particularly the way the question is phrased. Is it asking for the most important or the *first* response? Is it asking you for factual information, conceptual information, or nursing judgment? One of the most important principles in test taking is understanding precisely what the question is asking.

Strategy #2 Do not read extra meaning into the question.

In effective test construction, the stem is direct and to the point. The question asks for one particular response, and you should not read other information into the question. Reading into these questions, making interpretations, or searching for subtle hidden meanings is not advised. Your first action is to ask yourself, "What is the question asking?" Look for key words or phrases to help you understand. It is important to have the central point clearly in your mind before considering the distractors.

Determine what the question is really asking. Sometimes details are extraneous. Mentally underline important factors; pay attention to key terms and phrases. For example, do not misread *grams* as *milligrams*. Read the question as it is stated, not as you would like it to be stated. The questions will test your ability to analyze a clinical situation and to apply your nursing knowledge.

Do not look for a pattern in the answer key—there is none. For example, if you have already answered several consecutive questions with a #2, do not hesitate to answer the next question in sequence with a #2 if you think that is the right answer. Evaluate the possible answers in relation to the stem (the question), not to other answers. Choose the answer that best fits that question rather than an answer that sounds good by itself.

Strategy #3 Rephrase the question in your own words.

Another technique for assessing the stem and interpreting the question correctly is to rephrase the question so that it is very clear in your own mind. Rephrasing the stem of the question in your own language can assist you to read the question correctly and, in turn, choose the appropriate response. This is particularly important when you are faced with a difficult and/or confusing question.

> The nurse in the newborn nursery is unable to insert a tube into a newborn's stomach; she has met resistance with each attempt. Tracheoesophageal fistula with atresia is suspected. An important assessment is

To clearly understand the question, restate the condition in your own words: "With tracheoesophageal fistula, I know that there is a connection between the esophagus and the trachea." Then rephrase the question: "If there is an overflow of liquid into the larynx and trachea, what signs would I be likely to observe?" The answer is excessive drooling, choking and coughing during the feeding.

Placing the question in a framework that you understand will enable you to cut through extraneous data to the heart of the stem. Also, stating the question as a process—what assessment is important for a baby who has tracheoesophageal fistula with atresia—will allow you to follow the process to a logical conclusion (usually the correct answer). If possible, think of the correct answer before considering the distractors. If you do not know the answer, the following cues to working with distractors may prove helpful.

Strategy #4 When analyzing the distractors, isolate what is important in the answer alternatives from what is not important *relative to the question*.

Distractors are various alternatives chosen to be as close as possible to the right answer. In good test construction, all of the distractors are similar, should be feasible and reasonable, and should apply directly to the stem. Also, all of the distractors may contain correct information, but not be the right choice for the specific question that is asked. One method of helping you choose the correct answer is to ask yourself whether each alternative is true or false in relation to the stem.

> Which one of the following characteristics is not found with parents who abuse their children?
> 1. They have very low impulse control.   TRUE
> 2. They are socially isolated and lonely people.   TRUE
> 3. They have realistic expectations of their children.   FALSE
> 4. Often they were abused as children.   TRUE

Asking yourself which of the distractors is true or false is a shortcut method of answering the question. It forces you to keep looking at the stem. Otherwise you are trying to judge all of the choices at once. After you have completed the true-false process, remember to go back to the stem and ask yourself if your choice does, in fact, answer the question.

Strategy #5 After choosing the correct answer alternative and separating it from the distractors, go back to the stem and make sure your choice does, in fact, answer the question.

An answer alternative may be correct as it stands by itself, but if the question asks for the first nursing action, you need to separate *first* from *later* nursing interventions. Too many candidates fail to recheck the answer with the stem, and they answer the question incorrectly.

Strategy #6 Use the "process of elimination" technique.

Examine each alternative and ask yourself, "Is this answer right?" or "Is this answer logical?" Try to eliminate at least one or more distractors. If you can eliminate one or two distractors, it will be easier to identify the correct answer. The "process of elimination" is one of the most effective test-taking strategies.

Strategy #7 When answering a difficult question, utilize all of your knowledge.

When you come across a difficult question and you cannot immediately identify the answer, go back to your body of knowledge and draw on the information that you *do* know about the condition. Suppose you were asked a question about the most important equipment to have in the room when a client returns from surgery. You would know that brain surgery would require different equipment from lung surgery, especially when you consider the potential complications. Even if you don't know the answer immediately, by taking your time to analyze the situation, recalling the information you have learned about that condition, and applying this information to the specific situation presented in the question, you should be able to arrive at the correct answer. Also, if you are unfamiliar with the disease or disorder and cannot choose the right nursing action, try to generalize to other situations. Even though you don't know exactly what *to do*, you might know what *not* to do. The elimination of one distractor substantially increases the odds of your selecting the correct answer. To summarize the concept of generalizing, remember, if you don't know or recognize the specific condition, try to identify a general principle and apply it to that situation.

Strategy #8   The ability to guess correctly is both a skill and an art.

Because the NCLEX-PN exam requires you to answer each question before proceeding to the next one, you may, on occasion, have to guess. Guessing is an art in itself, and since you only have a 25% chance of guessing correctly, let's look at several strategies that may increase your odds.

1. Try to eliminate at least one (or more if possible) distractor, as this will increase your chances of guessing correctly.
2. Examine the distractors, and if one is the exact opposite of another (you know that unlimited fluid intake and restricted fluid intake cannot both be correct), choose the one that seems most logical.
3. Try to identify the underlying principle that supports the question. If you can answer the question, "What is this question trying to determine that I know?", you might then be able to guess the correct answer. This strategy is especially true with a psychosocial question.
4. Look at the way the alternatives are presented. Are two answers very close? Often when this occurs, the ability to discriminate will show evidence of judgment. Check to see if one, more than the other, is the best choice for the question.
5. Examine the alternatives for logic. Are some distractors just not logical? Are some distractors correct in themselves, but do not have anything to do with the question? If so, eliminate these and concentrate on the remaining alternatives.

Strategy #9   Choosing an answer from a "hunch."

During a test, you may come to a question and not know the answer immediately, but have an inner feeling or a hunch that a particular alternative is the right answer. Do you depend on this "hunch"? Current research supports that intuition is often correct, for such judgments are based on rapid subconscious connections in the brain. In other words, going through logical, rational steps is not the only way to arrive at the answer. Your stored knowledge, recall and experience can combine to assist you in arriving at the correct answer. So, if you have an initial hunch, go with it. **Do not** change the answer if, upon reflection, it just doesn't seem right.

On the other hand, if you re-read the question and note information you previously missed (for example, the age of the client or diagnosis related to diet), then you may feel it is appropriate to change your answer selection. With additional information or a definite conclusion, rather than a "feeling," it is a good test-taking strategy to change an answer. Remember, however, when taking the NCLEX CAT, you cannot go back to a prior question and change the answer. Before moving on to the next question, therefore, you must be careful to make certain of your choice.

Strategy #10 Choosing the most comprehensive answer.

The most comprehensive answer may be the best choice. For example, if two alternatives seem reasonable but one answer includes the other (i.e., it is more detailed, extends the first, or is more comprehensive), then this answer would be the best choice.

Guidelines for Answering Psychosocial Questions

The current test plan incorporates the psychosocial aspect of the illness, treatment, or client care plan. The psychosocial focus will be a central thread throughout the clinical areas: medical and surgical nursing, maternity and pediatric nursing. In other words, even though a question may be coded *medical* and deal with a client who has recently had a myocardial infarction, it is possible that the actual content of the question will relate to psychosocial nursing, rather than straight medical nursing. When you encounter psychosocial or communication-oriented questions, remember the following communication principles as guidelines for your answer choices.

1. *Responses that focus on feelings.* All clients at some time find it difficult to express their feelings whether they have a terminal illness, a new baby, a somatic illness, or are scheduled for elective surgery. Any nursing response that elicits these feelings is therapeutic, so listen and pay attention to client cues. When the client needs to discuss fears, concerns, or angry feelings, then encourage their expression. If a client states he is afraid of dying, encourage talking about fears of dying (be specific), not just fears (general response).

2. *Responses that are honest and direct.* It is important that the nurse be honest in her responses to encourage trust and build a therapeutic relationship. Dishonesty will never support trust and a firm relationship. So, if a client asks you a question, give an honest response.

3. *Responses that indicate acceptance of the client.* Accept the client where and how he is regardless of his condition or verbalizations. In fact, you should not reject the client, even if you could not accept his behavior.

4. *Responses that pick up or relate to cues.* Responding to an important cue is an essential therapeutic technique if the nurse is to focus on the client and maintain a goal-focused interaction. Respond to "feeling level" cues rather than "cognitive" or superficial cues from the client.

At the Test Session

Students who are relaxed and confident while taking tests have a distinct advantage over those who become extremely anxious when taking an important exam. Achieving the maximum testing effectiveness involves your mental attitude as well as your knowledge of specific testing techniques. The following suggestions will help you maximize your testing effectiveness.

1. *General readiness is a key to success.* Prepare the night before the test. Assemble the materials that you must take to the test site as specified in your instructions. Get a good night's rest. Don't stay up all night learning new material. Avoid the use of stimulants or depressants, either of which may affect your ability to think clearly during the test. Approach the test with confidence and the determination to do your best. Think positively and concentrate on all you *do* know rather than on what you think you *do not* know.

2. *On the day of the exam, get yourself together.* Eat a nutritious breakfast. Protein will provide needed energy. Allow ample time to travel to the testing site, including time to park, and to check in. Choose a location in the testing room where you are least likely to be distracted.

3. *Scoring well on the examination.* As you start your test, check the time periodically, and maintain a good rate of progression. Do not spend too much time on any one question so that you become anxious and immobilized. If you do not know the answer, choose one of the alternatives. Do not waste time by struggling with questions that totally perplex you.

Computer Testing Tips

1. Answer each question. If you don't recognize a correct answer among the four choices, use your test-taking skills or, if necessary, make your best guess.

2. Be certain of your answer selection before pressing the "Enter" key a second time to confirm your choice. You cannot change your answers to prior questions.

3. Take your time and carefully read the questions and answer choices. You have 5 hours and the maximum number of questions you will be asked is 205.

4. Do not become immobilized by any one question. Spending 5 to 10 minutes on a question will probably make you more nervous and less attentive as you proceed.

5. The test center will provide you with scratch paper and a pencil. Use them when you encounter questions that require calculations.

6. Take a nutritious snack and perhaps bottled water with you. At the test center you will be assigned a locker where you must leave your personal items. After 2 hours of testing, you will have a mandatory rest break of 10 minutes.

Summary

In summary, the information presented in this chapter provides you with guidelines and strategies, not absolutes. Always use your own judgment, knowledge, and nursing experience. These assets will serve you well in passing the NCLEX-PN. You have the background, education and knowledge to pass these exams. Let your own creative abilities come through. Be confident that you will pass and, in fact, you will.

Using Your Computer Disk

A 3.5" IBM compatible computer disk has been placed in an envelope inside the back cover of this book. The purposes of the practice disk include the following:

1. To provide you with simulated NCLEX CAT questions so you can rehearse taking NCLEX on the computer. This includes your reading questions (stem and distractors) as they will be displayed on the computer screen, rather than seeing them printed in a test booklet.

2. To enable you to become familiar with the computer procedures that you will follow when you take NCLEX. The computer keys used to display questions and select and confirm answers on your practice disk are the same designated keys you will use when you take NCLEX.

3. To give you useful feedback when you complete the simulated NCLEX test. You will be able to obtain a Performance Summary that will help you identify your strengths and weaknesses in terms of the Nursing Process, Client Needs, and Clinical Areas.

4. To identify the specific questions you missed so you can review the rationale for the correct answers. This will help you understand the principles that underlie the correct answers.

5. To enable you to experience additional practice. You will be able to erase the answers on your disk and retake the simulated test at a later date.

III

COMPREHENSIVE TESTS 1 & 2

COMPREHENSIVE TEST 1

1. An LVN who stops at an accident and renders health care is covered by the Good Samaritan Statute as long as he or she

    1 Only provides first aid treatment.
    2 Provides care they are legally prepared to administer.
    3 Does not cause further harm to the victim.
    4 Obtains permission from the victim to provide care.

2. Teaching a client about use of the insulin pump in preparation for discharge, the nurse will explain that it uses

    1 A combination of regular and Lente insulin delivered 2 times each day.
    2 Continuous delivery of small amounts of regular insulin.
    3 A predetermined dose established by a glucose tolerance test.
    4 A combination of NPH and regular insulin with NPH delivered in the morning.

3. A 24-year-old male client with no feeling or sensation in his lower extremities is in spinal shock. The nurse will be able to recognize that his condition is improving when

    1 The client's legs move.
    2 The client regains sensations but not motion in his upper extremities.
    3 Hyperreflexia occurs.
    4 The client's vital signs stabilize.

4. The type of diet that would be indicated for a child with cystic fibrosis is

    1 High calorie, high protein, low fat.
    2 Low carbohydrate, high protein, high fat.
    3 Low calorie, low fat, low protein.
    4 High carbohydrate, high fat, high protein.

5. A 4 year old with a diagnosis of possible epiglottitis is admitted to the pediatric unit. A *priority* nursing intervention will be to

    1 Avoid use of restraints.
    2 Keep the child in an upright position.
    3 Administer oxygen mist therapy.
    4 Monitor hydration status.

6. A client with a history of coronary artery disease asks for a snack between meals. The nurse asks him to list the snacks he likes that are allowed on his low fat, low sodium, low cholesterol diet. The nurse realizes that further dietary teaching is necessary when one of his choices is

    1 Buttermilk.
    2 A jam sandwich.
    3 An apple.
    4 Applesauce.

7. After a vaginal examination, the client's obstetrician tells her that she is at -1 station. When she asks the nurse what this means, the nurse tells her that station -1 means the presenting part of the fetus is

    1 In the false pelvis.
    2 At the level of the ischial spines.
    3 One cm above the level of the ischial spines.
    4 One cm below the level of the ischial spines.

8. In assessing the baby's position for delivery, the nurse knows that the *most favorable* position for delivery of an infant is a

    1 Transverse lie.
    2 Breech presentation.
    3 Right or left occiput posterior.
    4 Left or right occiput anterior.

9. The physician has ordered a footplate for a client on bedrest. The nurse understands that the purpose of this order is to

   1 Prevent pressure points on the feet.
   2 Protect the leg from skin breakdown.
   3 Prevent footdrop during immobilization.
   4 Maintain a 20-degree angle from thigh to bed.

10. The physician orders an upper GI series and a barium enema for an elderly female client. The client appears to be very anxious. The nurse can best help her cope with anxiety by

   1 Suggesting that she ask the doctor why he is ordering these tests.
   2 Diverting her attention by discussing a subject in which she is interested.
   3 Asking her if she would like to talk about the examination.
   4 Telling her not to worry because this type of x-ray doesn't hurt.

11. A male client, age 36, has a fractured hip and his physician has applied Buck's traction pre-operatively. The nursing assessment to ensure that there is adequate countertraction will include

   1 Weights hanging freely off the floor and bed.
   2 Ropes knotted to prevent them from moving through the pulleys.
   3 Checking that the client is pulled down on the bed, using the end board as a foot rest.
   4 Checking that the foot of the bed is elevated to provide countertraction.

12. Planning nursing care for the infant who is receiving phototherapy for hyperbilirubinemia, it is important to remember that bilirubin concentrations in excess of 15 to 18 mg/100 mL blood cause damage primarily to the

   1 Liver.
   2 Retina of the eyes.
   3 Kidneys.
   4 Brain.

13. When measuring a client for elastic hose, the nurse will measure the

   1 Leg length and ankle circumference while the client is standing.
   2 Ankle and calf circumference while the client is standing.
   3 Leg length after the client has been lying down.
   4 Ankle and calf circumference and leg length after the client has been lying down.

14. Following test results, the physician tells his client that malignancy may be present. She responds, "Oh, I know that nothing is wrong. I'm feeling much better." The client is using the defense mechanism of

   1 Reaction formation.
   2 Denial.
   3 Projection.
   4 Disbelieving.

15. The day after colostomy surgery, the client tells the nurse that she does not want to look at the stoma. The *best* way to handle this situation is to

   1 Urge her to look at the stoma so she can become accustomed to it.
   2 Consider this a normal response and respect her wishes.
   3 Notify the physician and ask him to talk with the client.
   4 Request that another person with an ostomy talk with her.

16. The nurse is assigned to care for a client pre-operatively, whose orders include Meperidine 25 mg IM at 7:30 AM. After checking the orders on the chart, the correct nursing action is to

   1 Call the anesthesiologist to double check the dosage, because it is in the lower range of normal.
   2 Use Z-track, not IM, method of injection to protect the injection site.

3 Follow orders and give the drug as prescribed.

4 Refuse to administer the medication because the dosage is incorrect.

17. A client returns from surgery following a hip replacement. An important postoperative nursing intervention for positioning this client is to

1 Maintain adduction of the affected hip.
2 Maintain abduction of the affected hip.
3 Avoid external rotation of the affected hip.
4 Keep her in Sims' position.

18. A 55-year-old client comes to an emergency department complaining of severe pain in his left big toe. A diagnosis of gout is made. In order to teach the client, the nurse should know that the primary medications for treatment of this condition are

1 Aspirin (ASA) and colchicine, U.S.P.
2 Colchicine, U.S.P and allopurinol, U.S.P.
3 Oxycodone hydrochloride and aspirin (Percodan) and allopurinol, U.S.P.
4 A corticosteroid and colchicine, U.S.P.

19. A client's IV is to run at 125 mL/hour. The IV administration set delivers 20 gtts/mL. At what rate will the nurse adjust the IV?

1 21 gtts/minute.
2 31 gtts/minute.
3 41 gtts/minute.
4 125 gtts/minute.

20. A young client, age 7, has been diagnosed as having sickle cell anemia. While teaching the mother about this condition, the nurse must understand the disease process. The *most accurate* description of sickle cell anemia is which one of the following?

1 It is similar to chronic anemia due to the inability to utilize iron.
2 Sickle-shaped red blood cells cause anemia.

3 Red blood cells that sickle under low oxygen tension cause the anemia.
4 Sickle cells combine with normal blood cells which results in anemia.

21. The nurse is at the bedside when a 9 year old has a seizure shortly after admission. The *first* action during the seizure is to

1 Call the physician immediately.
2 Place a tongue blade between the child's teeth.
3 Protect the child from injury by removing objects from the bed.
4 Observe the course of the seizure for future diagnosis.

22. A 3-month-old infant is brought to a clinic for a well-baby check-up. During data collection, the nurse learns that the infant's bottle is often propped in the crib because the baby wiggles a lot. Which of the following comments to the infant's parents would be *most therapeutic* for the nurse to make?

1 "It is probably a good idea to prop the bottle until you feel more comfortable holding the baby."
2 "It is not a good idea to prop the baby's bottle because she could choke on the formula."
3 "Do you have a fear of dropping the baby when you feed her?"
4 "You need to hold the baby when you are feeding her."

23. While explaining the side effects of oral contraceptives to a teenage client, the nurse will tell her that

1 There are no major side effects of the pill, so she won't have to worry.
2 The pill is so effective that she need not be concerned with the side effects.
3 If side effects occur, she should skip taking the pill for a few days, then resume.
4 Side effects may appear but these usually disappear within the first to third cycle.

24. When discussing family planning methods, the nurse should inform the couple that the *most effective* birth control method is

    1 Rhythm.
    2 Oral contraceptives
    3 Diaphragm.
    4 Chemical foam.

25. A 65-year-old male client with Parkinson's disease is being treated with L-Dopa. The nurse will know he understands the teaching principles when he says that he avoids foods rich in

    1 Vitamin B_{12}.
    2 Vitamin B_6.
    3 Vitamin A.
    4 Vitamin E.

26. A 42-year-old female client is admitted to a hospital with a suspected diagnosis of renal calculi. The physician has ordered an intravenous pyelogram. The *most important* preparation for this procedure is to

    1 Assess for shellfish allergy.
    2 Restrict fluids for 8 to 10 hours.
    3 Administer a laxative.
    4 Allow a light breakfast.

27. A female client comes to the maternity clinic and tells the nurse she has recently learned that she is pregnant. She is a vegetarian and asks the nurse how she can eat enough protein. One example the nurse can give her is that 2 to 3 ounces of meat equals

    1 One cup cottage cheese.
    2 One tablespoon peanut butter.
    3 One-half pint milk.
    4 One-half cup tofu or soybean cake.

28. A female client comes to the emergency room. The nurse's immediate assessment reveals that the client is bleeding profusely from a deep laceration on her left lower forearm. The *first* action is to

1 Apply a tourniquet just below the elbow.
2 Apply pressure directly over the wound.
3 Call for the physician to check the wound.
4 Place the client in shock position.

29. A 20-year-old client is admitted to a hospital with a diagnosis of acute schizophrenia. He is becoming more withdrawn and suspicious of other clients, and he constantly tries to argue with the nursing staff that several of the clients are "out to get him." The *best* nursing approach to this behavior is to

    1 Ignore the behavior and it will diminish.
    2 Disagree with him so that his fears will not be confirmed.
    3 Avoid disagreeing with him and get him involved with an activity.
    4 Reassure him that he will be protected from the other clients.

30. An 8-month-old male child is tentatively diagnosed as being mentally retarded. The parents have come to the hospital for further assessment and counseling. During the nurse's assessment, the observation that will help assess for mental retardation is that the child is unable to

    1 Sit unsupported for brief periods.
    2 Crawl short distances.
    3 Demonstrate a negative Babinski.
    4 Grasp a spoon and bring it to his mouth.

31. A 50-year-old female client is scheduled for a cholecystectomy. Following surgery, she has a T-tube in place and is returned to the surgical unit. Which position will ensure optimal functioning?

    1 Semi-Fowler's position.
    2 Prone position.
    3 High-Fowler's position.
    4 Sims' position.

32. The mother of a 1-month-old male infant brings him to a clinic for his well-baby check-

up. She asks the nurse when to start solid foods and what to feed him. The *most appropriate* response is to tell her to begin solid food at the age of

1   Two months with wheat cereal.
2   Five to 6 months with rice cereal.
3   Four to 6 months with fruits and vegetables.
4   Two to 3 months with bananas and applesauce.

33.   A 53-year-old male client has a history of deep vein thrombosis and his physician has ordered crystalline warfarin sodium (Coumadin). An important nutritional principle associated with this drug protocol is to instruct the client to

1   Avoid foods high in B vitamins.
2   Avoid spinach and green leafy vegetables.
3   Eat extra lettuce and dairy products.
4   Eat three meals a day and ensure it is a well-balanced diet.

34.   When charting the procedure for applying restraints to a client, the nurse will include

1   What the client says about the restraint.
2   Procedure utilized for applying the restraint.
3   Physician's orders regarding the restraint.
4   Condition of extremity following application.

35.   The type of client most at risk for complications when fecal impactions are removed would include those clients with a

1   CVA.
2   Diagnosis requiring long-term bedrest.
3   Permanent pacemaker.
4   Spinal cord injury.

36.   When the nurse identifies that the ECG pattern is not clearly displayed on the oscilloscope, the *first* intervention is to

1   Notify the charge nurse or physician.
2   Assess the client for excessive activity.
3   Assess if the client has any clinical changes.
4   Cleanse the skin with alcohol before applying new electrodes.

37.   When teaching a home care client the signs of pacemaker malfunction, the nurse should include

1   Increased urine output.
2   Regular, slow pulse.
3   Weakness, fatigue.
4   Disorientation.

38.   A female client has an admitting diagnosis of affective disorder–manic episode. She refuses to sit and eat with the other clients. The nurse understands that it is important for her to eat. Which of the following plans is *most appropriate* to adopt to accomplish this goal?

1   Allow her to eat in her room alone, because the nurse knows that the other clients on the unit disturb her.
2   Make available nutritional snacks and finger foods throughout the day, so she can eat when she wishes to do so.
3   Insist that she go to the dining room to sit and eat with other clients.
4   Tell her that the staff will have to tube feed her if she continues to refuse to eat.

39.   A female client has orders to take lithium regularly after being discharged from the hospital. Her serum level has been regulated at 1.4 mEq/l and she seems to be doing well. Which of the following is the *most important* discharge information to impart to the client and her family?

1   Side effects of gastrointestinal disturbance, thirst, polyuria, and muscle weakness may occur.
2   Drowsiness, tremors and slurred speech are early indications of lithium toxicity.

3 Hypothyroidism may occur and treatment should be instituted promptly.

4 She should not eat foods that have a high tyramine content, such as cheese, wine, liver, yeast, or alcohol.

40. The primary objective of treatment for clients with congestive heart failure is to

1 Reduce the workload of the heart.
2 Promote rest for the heart.
3 Reduce fluid retention.
4 Reduce circulating blood volume.

41. A client with the diagnosis of left-sided congestive heart failure complains of shortness of breath. The nurse understands that dyspnea associated with left-sided heart failure is due to

1 Accumulation of fluid in the alveoli.
2 Obstruction in the lungs by mucus.
3 Compression of the lungs by an enlarged heart.
4 Accumulation of blood in the left atrium.

42. A female client in congestive heart failure has orders that include administering 0.25 mg digoxin. When the nurse checks the client's pulse before giving the medication, the pulse rate is 58. The appropriate nursing action is to

1 Administer the digoxin.
2 Notify the charge nurse or physician.
3 Check the last dosage of digoxin.
4 Hold the dose of digoxin.

43. As the nurse is talking with a client, the client says she is afraid she is going to die. The *best* nursing response to this statement is

1 "Did the doctor tell you that you are going to die?"
2 "What makes you think you are going to die?"
3 "In this day of modern medicine, no one dies with your diagnosis."
4 "Tell me more about these fears."

44. The nurse instructs her pregnant client to immediately report any visual disturbances she may experience. The *best* rationale for this instruction is that the presence of this symptom indicates possible

1 Pre-eclampsia.
2 Increased intracranial pressure.
3 Glaucoma.
4 Medication toxicity.

45. The preoperative nursing care plan for a client scheduled for an iridectomy will include

1 Administering pilocarpine eye drops.
2 Administering cycloplegic eye drops.
3 Patching both eyes.
4 Patching the affected eye.

46. A client is lying comfortably on her back 30 minutes after receiving an epidural injection. The nurse checks fetal heart tones and the rate is 100 per minute. The *first* nursing action is to

1 Administer oxygen by mask as ordered PRN.
2 Turn the client onto her left side.
3 Recheck the fetal heart tones.
4 Take the client's blood pressure.

47. A new mother of a 1-month-old infant is concerned because the baby sleeps so much of the day. The nurse tells the mother that infants

1 Sleep all day and stay awake most of the night until they develop a regular routine.
2 Should have only one nap during the day.
3 Need at least 12 hours of sleep during every 24 hours.
4 Usually sleep about 20 of every 24 hours.

48. A 2-month-old female infant develops an ear infection. While administering ear drops, the appropriate technique is to place the baby

1 On her side and pull the ear auricle down and back.

2   On her side and administer the drops straight into her ear.

3   On her back and pull the ear auricle up and back.

4   In Fowler's position, then administer drops into her lower ear canal.

49.   When a child is at the toddler stage, it is most important for the mother to be aware of the

1   Safety hazards, such as poisons and medicine, which are within the child's reach.

2   Importance of mastering the autonomy stage of development.

3   Danger of the child eating dirt.

4   Possibility that the child may show jealousy toward other children.

50.   One of the primary goals of treatment for a client with acute glomerulonephritis would be to encourage

1   Fluid intake to restore fluid balance.

2   Complete bedrest during the acute phase.

3   A high protein diet to restore nutritional status.

4   Activity to facilitate diuresis.

51.   A client in the early stages of renal failure is given furosemide (Lasix). If the drug's action is effective, the nurse would expect a/an

1   Decrease in temperature.

2   Increase in pulse rate.

3   Decrease in blood pressure.

4   Increase in urinary output.

52.   A special diet is ordered for a client in renal failure. The main objective of diet control during the acute stage of renal failure is to

1   Increase the sodium intake to retain body fluids.

2   Reduce calories to decrease workload on the kidneys.

3   Reduce protein to protect kidney function.

4   Increase protein to encourage healing.

53.   A client with the diagnosis of dementia, Alzheimer's type, shuffles up to the station, crying and screaming, "Nobody cares if I live or die! You all hate me! You all hate me!" The *most therapeutic* response by the nurse is

1   "What makes you think we hate you?"

2   "You are always saying that and you know we all love you."

3   "Here is a cigarette. Now go in the dayroom and watch TV."

4   "You seem very upset. Let's take a walk and we can talk."

54.   Setting up a care plan for a male client with Alzheimer's disease, the nurse will include which one of the following goals?

1   Offer many choices for activities to keep him interested.

2   Allow him to function dependently on the nursing staff.

3   Instruct the staff to talk loudly to help him understand directions.

4   Provide a safe, structured environment.

55.   The nurse has just helped deliver a healthy baby boy, born precipitously in the emergency room. The *first* nursing action immediately after the birth is to

1   Keep the baby warm.

2   Gently suction the mouth, and, if necessary, the nose.

3   Place the baby on the mother's abdomen.

4   Slap the baby on his back to stimulate breathing.

56.   During a typical emergency delivery, which of the following principles best explains why the nurse will not cut the cord?

1   The physician is responsible for cutting the cord.

2   Cutting the cord under emergency conditions might lead to hemorrhage from the placenta.

3   Cutting the cord might lead to infection.

4   The nurse was not trained to perform the procedure.

57. Evaluating the home situation of a child whom the nurse suspects may be abused, the nurse knows that parents who abuse their children usually

    1 Have adequate impulse control.
    2 Do not have unreasonable expectations of their child.
    3 Care what happens to their child.
    4 Blame themselves for the injury.

58. During the immediate postoperative period following a tonsillectomy for a 4 year old, the nurse would position the child in

    1 Semi-Fowler's.
    2 Sims'.
    3 Trendelenburg's.
    4 Supine.

59. An AIDS client asks the nurse whether he should tell his partner that he has AIDS. The *best* nursing response is

    1 "Do you think you contracted AIDS from your partner?"
    2 "What are you thinking you should do?"
    3 "No, I don't think you should tell him."
    4 "Perhaps you should discuss this with your doctor."

60. The nurse is assigned to give a gastrostomy tube feeding. Aspirating the gastric contents, the residual measures 120 mL. The nursing intervention is to

    1 Hold the next feeding and discard the residual.
    2 Administer the feeding together with the residual.
    3 Administer the feeding and discard the residual.
    4 Hold the feeding and return the residual.

61. A 2-year-old client has a fracture of his right femur. Observing whether Bryant's traction is properly assembled, the nurse will expect to see the

    1 Moleskin taut and placed on either side of the lower leg to provide traction.
    2 Weights attached to a pin which is inserted in the femur.
    3 Pin site and weights aligned in a horizontal position.
    4 Weights attached to skin traction and hung freely from the crib.

62. During the postoperative period following cardiac surgery, the client complains of incisional pain. The nurse notes that the client's respirations are shallow but unlabored. The *first* intervention is to

    1 Encourage the client to drink more fluids.
    2 Start oxygen at 10 L/minute via nasal prongs as ordered.
    3 Administer the ordered pain medication.
    4 Encourage the client to take slow, deep breaths.

63. A client with the diagnosis of schizophrenia tells the nurse that there is nothing wrong with her—it's the fault of her family that she is in the hospital and that they are out to get her. This defense mechanism is called

    1 Introjection.
    2 Denial.
    3 Projection.
    4 Reaction-formation.

64. The nurse observes a schizophrenic female client sitting, staring into space, occasionally saying something like "Is the world coming to an end?" The nurse's understanding of a comment like this is that the client is

    1 Experiencing paranoid ideation so she is afraid of everything.
    2 Having difficulty telling the difference between her own wishes and fears and what is real.
    3 Really asking the nurse for reassurance that she is going to be safe.
    4 Expressing a typical catatonic form of speech.

65. A new mother is now 36 hours postpartum and has an oral temperature of 38.3° C (101° F). Appropriate nursing assessment includes which of the following nursing actions?

 1 Ask the client if she would like warm soaks to her breasts.
 2 Check the lochia for odor and color.
 3 Check the height of the fundus.
 4 Ask the client if she has any pain.

66. The nurse is assigned to observe a client closely for signs of magnesium toxicity following an IV of 4 gm magnesium sulfate in 250 mL 0.5% D/W. The first indication of this condition is

 1 Decreased urine output.
 2 Peripheral vasodilation.
 3 Extreme thirst.
 4 Change in Babinski reflex.

67. Which of the paired clients would the team leader assign a new graduate LVN to care for?

 1 A recent postop client with abdominal surgery and a client admitted with infection of unknown origin.
 2 An AIDS client and a client with lobar pneumonia.
 3 A diabetic client for evaluation and a client with COPD.
 4 A client receiving chemotherapy and a client with an upper respiratory infection.

68. For a diagnosis of viral pneumonia in a 6 month old, the nursing diagnosis is fluid deficit. The *best* method of ensuring a proper fluid balance during the acute stage of the infant's illness is to administer

 1 Half-strength formula.
 2 Water by nasogastric tube.
 3 IV infusion of 5% dextrose and water.
 4 Full-strength formula.

69. A goal in the care plan for a 9 month old with pneumonia is to facilitate breathing. The *best* position to achieve this goal is

 1 Trendelenburg's.
 2 Semi-Fowler's.
 3 Knee-chest.
 4 Sims'.

70. The nursing staff of a psychiatric unit planned an all-day outing. Many of the clients were on large doses of phenothiazines. A nursing action important to implement prior to the outing is to

 1 Obtain sunscreen and hats for the clients.
 2 Avoid excessive stimuli so the clients don't get out of control.
 3 Obtain a first-aid kit, because psychiatric clients are accident prone.
 4 Bring foods that do not contain caffeine or tyramine such as cheese, cola, coffee, or chocolate.

71. The nurse is assigned a client with the diagnosis of diabetes insipidus. Considering this diagnosis, the highest priority for the initial assessment of this client would be to assess

 1 Urine sugar and acetone.
 2 Neurological status.
 3 Urine output with specific gravity.
 4 Temperature, pulse and respiration.

72. A 23-year old female client, following an automobile accident, was placed in skeletal traction for a fractured femur. In the assessment of this client, one of the nurse's first concerns will be to assess for

 1 Skin excoriation.
 2 Placement of the bandages and tape.
 3 Proper alignment.
 4 Pressure points.

73. A newborn shows signs of jaundice, and the lab value for bilirubin shows a total bilirubin

of 15.0. The physician orders a continuous bili light. An important nursing intervention when an infant undergoes phototherapy is to

1 Cover the eyes with eye patches to prevent retinal damage.
2 Dress the infant to prevent chilling.
3 Isolate the infant to prevent cross-contamination.
4 Avoid handling the infant so as not to interfere with the treatment.

74. A 78-year-old female client has developed a pressure ulcer on her sacrum. The nurse teaches the nursing assistant that the *most appropriate* nursing intervention to prevent the ulcer from developing further is to

1 Place the client on a sheepskin pad.
2 Turn the client from side to side frequently—at least every 2 hours.
3 Place the client in a whirlpool bath daily.
4 Do passive range-of-motion at least 2 times daily.

75. The nurse is applying a wet-to-dry dressing on a client's pressure ulcer. Before applying the wet dressing, the nurse wrings out the excessive moisture. The rationale for this action is to

1 Prevent the dressing from leaking on the bed clothes.
2 Allow the dressing to dry between changes to trap the necrotic material.
3 Enable the dressing to dry on the ulcer to promote healing.
4 Allow the dressing to dry in 2 hours.

76. If the nurse has assessed a severe allergic reaction following the initiation of a blood transfusion, the *first* action is to

1 Relieve the symptoms and make the client comfortable.
2 Call the physician.
3 Slow the rate of infusion.
4 Stop the transfusion.

77. Dilantin is ordered to control a 10 year old's seizures. While teaching her mother about the medication, one of the side effects to emphasize is

1 Mood disturbances.
2 Drowsiness.
3 Bleeding gums.
4 Mild ataxia.

78. The physician orders a client to be out of bed in a tilted wheelchair following hip replacement surgery. The nurse requests the nursing assistant's help and explains to the NA that before helping the client out of bed, it is important to

1 Dangle the client on the edge of the bed before moving her to the wheelchair.
2 Ask the client if she feels strong enough to get out of bed.
3 Avoid positions with 30-degree to 45-degree flexion.
4 Not allow the client to bear weight on the affected hip.

79. When an elderly female client is diagnosed with depression, the risk of suicide is always of primary importance and concern to the nurse. Which one of the following behaviors indicates an increased risk of suicide?

1 The client's attitude and demeanor suddenly appear to be calm, satisfied, and suggest that everything will be all right.
2 The client's energy level is low and she appears to be more depressed now than upon admission.
3 The client begins to talk about leaving the hospital and what she will do to keep busy.
4 The client begins to express a great deal of anger toward the staff.

80. The nurse is assigned to care for a depressed client. The activity that is *most appropriate* for this client is

1 Participation in group therapy.
2 Helping another client make a cake.

3   Emptying the wastebaskets on the unit.

4   Learning to knit a sweater.

81.   A male client's hematocrit fell drastically following a GI bleed so the physician ordered 6 units of packed cells. The *most important* safety factor prior to starting the blood transfusion is to

1   Check the temperature of the blood.

2   Obtain the total number of units of blood that has been cross-matched.

3   Identify the type of IV controller being used for administration.

4   Check the blood bank number on the transfusion record and blood bag.

82.   A client with a long history of peptic ulcer disease is scheduled for a gastrectomy. One of the preoperative medications the nurse is preparing is atropine sulfate. A side effect often experienced by clients receiving this drug is

1   Dry mouth.

2   Urinary urgency.

3   Bradycardia.

4   Constricted pupils.

83.   During the postoperative period following abdominal surgery, the client will require airway suctioning. The nurse should keep the suction catheter in the airway for only 10 to 15 seconds in order to prevent

1   Tissue trauma.

2   Increased mucus.

3   Hypoxemia.

4   Infection.

84.   Following a client's gastrectomy, the nurse must explain the need for lifetime replacement of

1   Hydrochloric acid.

2   Antacids.

3   Vitamin B_{12}.

4   Gastric acid.

85.   There is an order to perform the credé procedure on a male client every 6 hours. "Credé" is a term used for a

1   Type of French catheter.

2   Surgical procedure for urinary diversion.

3   Manual method of expelling urine from the bladder.

4   Method of early bowel training following surgery.

86.   A client has a chest tube connected to two-bottle water-seal suction. The purpose of water in the second bottle is to

1   Provide humidity for the oxygen.

2   Maintain a closed system so air cannot enter the pleural space.

3   Provide a sterile environment for drainage.

4   Provide for an accurate means to measure drainage.

87.   Following lobectomy surgery, a nursing measure that assists in preventing thrombophlebitis is

1   Providing footboard walking.

2   Frequent massaging of both legs.

3   Gatching the knee of the bed.

4   Supporting the popliteal area with pillows.

88.   A physician orders an IV of D_5W with 3000 mL to run over 24 hours. How many calories is the client receiving?

1   200 calories.

2   400 calories.

3   600 calories.

4   1200 calories.

89.   Immediate postoperative nursing interventions for an above-the-knee amputation will include

1 Changing the dressing as necessary.

2 Keeping a tourniquet at the client's bedside.

3 Turning the client on his abdomen to prevent contractures.

4 Maintaining the client's position on the affected side to lessen chances of hemorrhage.

90. The nurse will help a child with acute glomerulonephritis follow a diet regimen of

1 Low sodium, low calorie.

2 Low potassium, low protein.

3 Fluid intake of 1000 mL/24 hours.

4 Low calcium, low potassium.

COMPREHENSIVE TEST 1
Answers with Rationale

1. (2) Good Samaritan laws cover nurses who provide care and practice using the standards of nursing as guidelines. The Nurse Practice Act is the legal guideline that should be followed when providing care to accident victims.

   Nursing Process: Planning
   Client Needs: Health Promotion and Maintenance
   Clinical Area: Medical Nursing

2. (2) The insulin pump mimics the release of insulin by the pancreas in a continuous delivery of fixed small amounts of regular insulin. It is capable of delivering larger doses before meals.

   Nursing Process: Implementation
   Client Needs: Safe, Effective Care Environment
   Clinical Area: Medical Nursing

3. (3) Reflex activity begins to return below the level of injury because of automatic activity inherent in nervous tissue.

   Nursing Process: Evaluation
   Client Needs: Physiological Integrity
   Clinical Area: Medical Nursing

4. (1) High calorie and protein intake will support growth and weight gain. A low fat diet is encouraged because the fat is poorly digested. Pancreatic enzymes are replaced and given with meals to assist with the digestion and absorption of fat.

   Nursing Process: Implementation
   Client Needs: Physiological Integrity
   Clinical Area: Pediatric Nursing

5. (2) An upright position maintains a patent airway. These children usually sit upright, leaning forward with their tongue protruding. The other interventions will be carried out, but airway maintenance is a priority.

   Nursing Process: Implementation
   Client Needs: Safe, Effective Care Environment
   Clinical Area: Pediatric Nursing

6. (1) Buttermilk contains large amounts of fat and must be avoided. Fruits and whole grains are encouraged.

   Nursing Process: Evaluation
   Client Needs: Health Promotion and Maintenance
   Clinical Area: Medical Nursing

7. (3) Station is the degree to which the presenting part has descended into the pelvis—the relationship between the presenting part and the ischial spine. The fetus moves from above to below the level of the ischial spines.

   Nursing Process: Implementation
   Client Needs: Health Promotion and Maintenance
   Clinical Area: Maternity Nursing

8. (4) Left or right occiput anterior (LOA and ROA) are the most favorable positions for delivery. Breech, where the buttocks or lower extremities are the presenting part, is a difficult delivery position and a transverse lie necessitates delivery by C-section.

   Nursing Process: Data Collection
   Client Needs: Physiological Integrity
   Clinical Area: Maternity Nursing

9. (3) A footplate placed against the client's feet will prevent footdrop during immobilization. It will not prevent pressure points on the feet or protect the skin. A footplate will not assist in maintaining a certain angle from thigh to bed.

> *Nursing Process:* Planning
> *Client Needs:* Physiological Integrity
> *Clinical Area:* Medical Nursing

10. (3) One of the best methods of dealing with anxiety is discussing these feelings. Asking the client to talk about the examination will give her an opportunity to verbalize her fears and will help alleviate her anxiety. Diverting her attention will not solve the problem, nor will telling her not to worry; this would, in fact, be nontherapeutic, as it is false reassurance.

> *Nursing Process:* Implementation
> *Client Needs:* Psychosocial Integrity
> *Clinical Area:* Psychiatric Nursing

11. (1) Weights must hang freely off the floor and bed to ensure countertraction. Ropes should be securely knotted, but they must move freely through pulleys. The client should not be pulled down in bed, because this position will negate the effect of the traction.

> *Nursing Process:* Data Collection
> *Client Needs:* Safe, Effective Care Environment
> *Clinical Area:* Surgical Nursing

12. (4) The brain is highly affected by increased levels of unconjugated bilirubin, which can cause brain damage through the process called kernicterus. Concentrations above 13 to 15 mg/100 mL are considered abnormal elevations.

> *Nursing Process:* Planning
> *Client Needs:* Physiological Integrity
> *Clinical Area:* Pediatric Nursing

13. (4) The leg length and ankle and calf circumferences should be measured after the client has been lying down. This causes the peripheral edema to be minimal and ensures that the hose fit snugly to offer maximum support.

> *Nursing Process:* Implementation
> *Client Needs:* Safe, Effective Care Environment
> *Clinical Area:* Medical Nursing

14. (2) Denial is the refusal to face reality. Denial of illness or, in this case, the possibility of malignancy, is a common way to protect oneself. Reaction formation and projection are not the appropriate defense mechanisms and disbelieving is not a defense mechanism.

> *Nursing Process:* Evaluation
> *Client Needs:* Psychosocial Integrity
> *Clinical Area:* Psychiatric Nursing

15. (2) So soon after surgery, this is considered a normal response. It is appropriate to respect the client's wishes at this time and in this way until she is ready to deal with the stoma. It may also be helpful to have another person with a stoma talk with the client, but this would be appropriate later in the acceptance process.

> *Nursing Process:* Implementation
> *Client Needs:* Psychosocial Integrity
> *Clinical Area:* Psychiatric Nursing

16. (3) This is a correct dosage for a preoperative medication, so the nurse would administer the drug as prescribed. The Z-track method would normally not be used for this drug, but for injection of iron in order to protect the tissue.

> *Nursing Process:* Implementation
> *Client Needs:* Safe, Effective Care Environment
> *Clinical Area:* Surgical Nursing

17. (2) For hip replacement surgery, it is important to keep the operative leg in abduction to prevent flexion. Frequent positioning is also important, but the bed should not be elevated more than 30 to 45 degrees.

> *Nursing Process:* Implementation
> *Client Needs:* Safe, Effective Care Environment
> *Clinical Area:* Surgical Nursing

18. (2) The medication of choice to reduce inflammation is colchicine, U.S.P. PO or even IV every hour for 8 hours until pain subsides; and allopurinol, U.S.P. to decrease uric acid levels. The action and side effects of these medications should be conveyed to the client. An analgesic may also be given for pain.

> *Nursing Process:* Planning
> *Client Needs:* Physiological Integrity
> *Clinical Area:* Medical Nursing

19. (3) The general formula to complete this calculation is

$$\frac{\text{Volume infused x drops/mL}}{\text{Time for infusing in minutes}} = \text{Drops/min}$$

$$\frac{125 \times 20}{60} = 41 \text{ Drops/min}$$

> *Nursing Process:* Implementation
> *Client Needs:* Safe, Effective Care Environment
> *Clinical Area:* Medical Nursing

20. (3) The client's red blood cells are not always sickled but become this way when certain conditions cause deoxygenation, such as exertion, infection and dehydration. These deformed cells then become entangled with each other and obstruct blood flow.

> *Nursing Process:* Data Collection
> *Client Needs:* Physiological Integrity
> *Clinical Area:* Pediatric Nursing

21. (3) The primary nursing action during a seizure is to protect the client from physical injury by removing objects that could harm him during the convulsions.

> *Nursing Process:* Implementation
> *Client Needs:* Safe, Effective Care Environment
> *Clinical Area:* Pediatric Nursing

22. (3) Before explaining the importance of holding the infant to develop the parent-child relationship, it is necessary to find out how the parents are feeling and to identify fears. All of the other responses close off communication.

> *Nursing Process:* Collecting Data
> *Client Needs:* Psychosocial Integrity
> *Clinical Area:* Pediatric Nursing

23. (4) There are expected side effects, such as weight gain, nausea and vomiting, but these usually disappear after a few months. There are some potential major side effects that the client should be told about so she can recognize them if they occur. She should not skip taking the pill for a few days, because she could become pregnant.

> *Nursing Process:* Implementation
> *Client Needs:* Health Promotion and Maintenance
> *Clinical Area:* Maternity Nursing

24. (2) Oral contraceptives are the most effective form of birth control except, of course, abstinence or sterilization.

> *Nursing Process:* Implementation
> *Client Needs:* Health Promotion and Maintenance
> *Clinical Area:* Maternity Nursing

25. (2) Foods rich in B_6 block the desired effects of L-Dopa; therefore, they need to be omitted from the diet. Examples of foods to be avoided include meat, especially organ meats,

whole-grain cereals, peanuts, and wheat germ.

Nursing Process: Evaluation
Client Needs: Health Promotion and Maintenance
Clinical Area: Medical Nursing

26. (1) It is important to assess for shellfish allergy to determine if the client is allergic to iodine, because the dye will contain this substance. Fluid restriction is observed; a laxative is ordered, but identifying a possible allergic reaction is the most important.

Nursing Process: Data Collection
Client Needs: Physiological Integrity
Clinical Area: Medical Nursing

27. (1) One cup of cottage cheese contains as much protein as a 2 or 3 ounce serving of meat. One cup of tofu or soybean or ¼ cup peanut butter each equal 1 serving of meat.

Nursing Process: Planning
Client Needs: Health Promotion and Maintenance
Clinical Area: Maternity Nursing

28. (2) The first action is to apply direct pressure to the wound. If the bleeding continues, additional actions must be taken. They include placing the client in shock position and perhaps applying a tourniquet.

Nursing Process: Implementation
Client Needs: Safe, Effective Care Environment
Clinical Area: Medical Nursing

29. (3) This is the best choice. The nurse should avoid power struggles, as this increases anxiety. Answer (4) is nontherapeutic; it will reinforce suspicions about other clients.

Nursing Process: Implementation
Client Needs: Psychosocial Integrity
Clinical Area: Psychiatric Nursing

30. (1) At 6 months of age, a child should be sitting with minimal support. Often, retarded children have flaccid muscles and loose joints which prevent the attainment of simple developmental milestones. The ability to sit is one of the most important milestones.

Nursing Process: Data Collection
Client Needs: Psychosocial Integrity
Clinical Area: Pediatric Nursing

31. (1) Initially a low-Fowler's position, then a semi-Fowler's position is encouraged, but not high-Fowler's. The objective is to facilitate drainage, as well as allow a position of comfort for the client.

Nursing Process: Planning
Client Needs: Physiological Integrity
Clinical Area: Surgical Nursing

32. (2) Waiting 5 to 6 months to start solid food allows the baby's GI tract to mature. Infants are least allergic to rice cereal, so it is preferable to start feedings with this food.

Nursing Process: Implementation
Client Needs: Health Promotion and Maintenance
Clinical Area: Pediatric Nursing

33. (2) The antagonist for Coumadin is vitamin K. Therefore, foods high in vitamin K, such as spinach, should be avoided.

Nursing Process: Planning
Client Needs: Health Promotion and Maintenance
Clinical Area: Medical Nursing

34. (4) Evaluation of the effects of the restraint is important to chart. Procedure is not relevant and what the client says may or may not be appropriate. Physician orders are already charted (restraints cannot be applied without orders), so the nurse would not chart them again.

Nursing Process: Implementation
Client Needs: Safe, Effective Care
Environment
Clinical Area: Psychosocial Integrity

35.   (4)   Spinal cord injured clients can develop a
vagal response from manual removal of feces,
which could result in bradycardia. The other
diagnoses would not be affected.

Nursing Process: Planning
Client Needs: Physiological Integrity
Clinical Area: Medical Nursing

36.   (2)   Excessive activity is termed artifact and
depicted on the screen as a very erratic
rhythm. If activity is not the cause or if any
clinical changes have occurred, then the nurse
would immediately notify the charge nurse.

Nursing Process: Implementation
Client Needs: Safe, Effective Care
Environment
Clinical Area: Medical Nursing

37.   (3)   Weakness and fatigue are two symptoms
that indicate hypoxia to tissues and a pacemaker malfunction. Increased urine output
and disorientation may need to be checked
out, but do not indicate pacemaker malfunction.

Nursing Process: Implementation
Client Needs: Health Promotion and
Maintenance
Clinical Area: Medical Nursing

38.   (2)   This client is expending a great deal of
energy caused by her manic disorder, so it is
very important that she ingest adequate nutrients. Nutritional snacks and finger foods
throughout the day will provide food for her
while she is moving about the unit. No mentally disturbed client should eat alone in their
room, because it is not safe. To insist that the
client sit in the dining room is unrealistic—

she may find it difficult to sit for even a short
while. Threatening her with tube feeding is
nontherapeutic.

Nursing Process: Planning
Client Needs: Safe, Effective Care
Environment
Clinical Area: Psychiatric Nursing

39.   (2)   Most important is that the client and
family be aware of lithium toxicity; these
symptoms are indicators of this condition.
Answer (1) includes expected side effects.
Hypothyroidism may be a side effect, but it is
not immediately critical. Foods with high tyramine content should not be eaten if one is taking MAO inhibitors.

Nursing Process: Planning
Client Needs: Health Promotion and
Maintenance
Clinical Area: Psychiatric Nursing

40.   (1)   Reducing the workload of the heart is the
most comprehensive answer and to accom-
plish this, the nurse would promote rest and
implement interventions that would reduce
fluid retention. Reducing fluid retention helps
reduce the circulating blood volume.

Nursing Process: Planning
Client Needs: Physiological Integrity
Clinical Area: Medical Nursing

41.   (1)   In left-sided failure there is increased
pulmonary pressure and congestion. Dyspnea
is caused by congestion in the pulmonary cir-
cuit due to the inability of the left side of the
heart to accommodate pulmonary vein input.
The accumulation of fluid in the alveoli causes
major pulmonary symptoms.

Nursing Process: Data Collection
Client Needs: Physiological Integrity
Clinical Area: Medical Nursing

42. (4) The action of digitalis is to slow the heart rate. When a client's pulse is under 60, the nursing action is to *not administer* or hold the drug. The nurse would then notify the physician.

> *Nursing Process:* Implementation
> *Client Needs:* Safe, Effective Care Environment
> *Clinical Area:* Medical Nursing

43. (2) This is an assessment response so that the nurse may gather more data concerning how she reached this conclusion. Answer (4) is nonspecific and while it opens communication, the nurse should first gather more data before discussing the fear of dying. Asking what the physician said is not relevant. Answer (3) is false reassurance, and, in addition, is not accurate.

> *Nursing Process:* Data Collection
> *Client Needs:* Psychosocial Integrity
> *Clinical Area:* Psychiatric Nursing

44. (1) If just visual disturbances are present, it may indicate pre-eclampsia, and the physician should be notified so the client may be closely followed. Visual disturbances, blurring, or even blindness can be caused by edema of the retina from a severe form of eclampsia.

> *Nursing Process:* Planning
> *Client Needs:* Physiological Integrity
> *Clinical Area:* Maternity Nursing

45. (1) Pilocarpine acts directly on the myoneural junction; it constricts the pupils and forces the iris away from the trabecular, allowing fluid to escape. Cycloplegic drops are given preoperatively with a cataract to paralyze the ciliary muscle, and postoperatively to relax the ciliary muscle with an iridectomy.

> *Nursing Process:* Planning
> *Client Needs:* Physiological Integrity
> *Clinical Area:* Surgical Nursing

46. (2) This form of regional anesthesia may cause transitory fetal bradycardia. The first nursing action is to turn the client onto her left side, shifting the weight of the fetus off the inferior vena cava. If the condition does not change after repositioning, then administer oxygen, as ordered. The next two actions would be to check the fetal heart rate and the mother's blood pressure.

> *Nursing Process:* Implementation
> *Client Needs:* Safe, Effective Care Environment
> *Clinical Area:* Maternity Nursing

47. (4) Young infants sleep about 20 hours a day. They are usually awake to eat, gurgle a little, and then go back to sleep. Napping during the day and only sleeping 12 hours a day occurs much later.

> *Nursing Process:* Implementation
> *Client Needs:* Health Promotion and Maintenance
> *Clinical Area:* Maternity Nursing

48. (1) The appropriate technique is to pull the ear auricle down and back so that the ear drops fall into the ear canal. The infant may be on her side or back with her head turned for this procedure. This question asks for technique, so answer (1) is more appropriate. If the nurse is administering ear drops to adults, the procedure is to pull the ear auricle up and back.

> *Nursing Process:* Implementation
> *Client Needs:* Safe, Effective Care Environment
> *Clinical Area:* Pediatric Nursing

49. (1) When there is a choice, safety is always considered first. In this question, safety hazards such as poisons, drugs or detergents are important to place out of reach or in locked cupboards so they cannot be found by a curious toddler. A toddler is in the stage of auton-

omy versus shame and doubt according to Erikson, but this is not a safety issue. Eating dirt may indicate a nutritional deficiency, but it is not as critical as ensuring home safety.

Nursing Process: Planning
Client Needs: Health Promotion and Maintenance
Clinical Area: Pediatric Nursing

50. (2) Bedrest during the acute phase will protect the kidneys from added stress. Activity may increase urinary abnormalities as well as facilitate diuresis. When the kidneys recover, fluid balance and mild hypertension will be alleviated. The diet should be low, not high, protein to protect the kidneys from processing protein waste products.

Nursing Process: Planning
Client Needs: Physiological Integrity
Clinical Area: Medical Nursing

51. (4) Lasix actually increases blood flow to the kidneys, thereby increasing the production of urine. This drug will not have a major effect on the other vital signs.

Nursing Process: Evaluation
Client Needs: Physiological Integrity
Clinical Area: Medical Nursing

52. (3) A low protein diet is important because damaged kidneys may not be able to eliminate waste products of protein digestion. Protein, not calories, affects the kidneys in terms of processing waste products.

Nursing Process: Planning
Client Needs: Physiological Integrity
Clinical Area: Medical Nursing

53. (4) The nurse acknowledges the client and his feelings without focusing directly on them. Answer (1) asks for an analysis of feelings. Answer (2) is making light of the client's feelings. Answer (3) is ignoring the problem.

Nursing Process: Implementation
Client Needs: Psychosocial Integrity
Clinical Area: Psychiatric Nursing

54. (4) Because dementia clients may have poor judgment, it is important to maintain a safe environment. Structure is also important, because it will decrease the anxiety. The other possibilities are incorrect: many choices will create anxiety; the nursing goal is to help him function as independently as possible; and, it is the mental capacity that is affected, not senses, such as hearing or vision.

Nursing Process: Planning
Client Needs: Safe, Effective Care Environment
Clinical Area: Psychiatric Nursing

55. (2) The highest priority action is to establish a patent airway, so the nurse would wipe off mucus or, if necessary, suction the mouth and then the nose. After this, the nurse would wrap the baby to keep it warm and place the baby on the mother's abdomen. The nurse would not slap the baby on the back to stimulate breathing, because it may cause the baby to aspirate.

Nursing Process: Implementation
Client Needs: Safe, Effective Care Environment
Clinical Area: Maternity Nursing

56. (3) The rationale for not cutting the cord following an emergency delivery is that lack of sterility could lead to infection. Hemorrhage might also occur, but not from the placenta. Answers (1) and (4) are not relevant principles to explain why the cord should not be cut.

Nursing Process: Planning
Client Needs: Safe, Effective Care Environment
Clinical Area: Maternity Nursing

57. (3) Parents who abuse their children often care very much about them, but they have very little understanding of how to deal with crises and the child's frustrating behavior. They have low impulse control (1) and unreasonable expectations (2) of their child.

> *Nursing Process:* Evaluation
> *Client Needs:* Psychosocial Integrity
> *Clinical Area:* Pediatric Nursing

58. (2) Prone or Sims' position is most appropriate to facilitate drainage of secretions and prevent aspiration. After the child is fully awake, he may be placed in semi-Fowler's position.

> *Nursing Process:* Implementation
> *Client Needs:* Safe, Effective Care Environment
> *Clinical Area:* Surgical Nursing

59. (2) The most therapeutic response is to maintain open communication and assist the client to answer his own question. Giving advice in this situation is nontherapeutic because it ultimately closes off communication. Referring the problem to the physician also closes communication.

> *Nursing Process:* Implementation
> *Client Needs:* Psychosocial Integrity
> *Clinical Area:* Psychiatric Nursing

60. (4) If there is more than 50 to 100 mL of gastric contents as residual, the next feeding should be held until the residual diminishes. The residual should be returned to the stomach to prevent fluid and electrolyte imbalance.

> *Nursing Process:* Implementation
> *Client Needs:* Safe, Effective Care Environment
> *Clinical Area:* Medical Nursing

61. (4) Bryant's traction is a form of skin traction and, therefore, does not require a pin insertion. Moleskin is frequently used as the stabilizing material for traction application. The weights must hang freely from the crib to maintain alignment and decrease the fracture.

> *Nursing Process:* Evaluation
> *Client Needs:* Safe, Effective Care Environment
> *Clinical Area:* Pediatric Nursing

62. (4) The first nursing action, before administering pain medication, is to encourage the client to relax and take slow, deep breaths. Slow breathing helps to reduce stress and pain, which may be caused as much by fear as actual incisional pain.

> *Nursing Process:* Implementation
> *Client Needs:* Safe, Effective Care Environment
> *Clinical Area:* Surgical Nursing

63. (3) The client is using projection when she blames her family, saying they are out to get her. Projection is placing the blame for one's difficulties on others; it is an indicator of paranoia.

> *Nursing Process:* Data Collection
> *Client Needs:* Psychosocial Integrity
> *Clinical Area:* Psychiatric Nursing

64. (2) A central problem in schizophrenia is difficulty in reality-testing, where the client often cannot tell the difference between what is real and what is not. This statement is not necessarily paranoid ideation, so answer (1) is incorrect; answer (3) is an interpretation of what the client is saying, thus incorrect. This question is not a catatonic form of speech. Most catatonics are mute or confused in their speech.

> *Nursing Process:* Data Collection
> *Client Needs:* Psychosocial Integrity
> *Clinical Area:* Psychiatric Nursing

65. (2) An increase in temperature might indicate an infection, so the first nursing assessment will be to check the lochia. The height of the fundus does not directly relate to an increase in temperature. Engorged breasts might be accompanied by an increase in temperature, but the highest priority is to assess for infection.

> *Nursing Process:* Data Collection
> *Client Needs:* Safe, Effective Care Environment
> *Clinical Area:* Maternity Nursing

66. (3) The first sign that the nurse will observe is probably extreme thirst. There will also be a loss of the patellar, not the Babinski, reflex. There will also be decreased urine output; however, this may be a later sign.

> *Nursing Process:* Evaluation
> *Client Needs:* Physiological Integrity
> *Clinical Area:* Maternity Nursing

67. (3) Assigning paired clients where there is the least chance of cross-contamination is the goal of this assignment. Pairing the diabetic and COPD clients, though not an ideal combination, would be the safest nursing practice.

> *Nursing Process:* Planning
> *Client Needs:* Health Promotion and Maintenance
> *Clinical Area:* Medical Nursing

68. (3) One of the dangers of high temperatures in young children is dehydration. It is critical to restore fluid balance, so IV infusion is the preferred treatment. Dextrose and water is a hypotonic solution that causes cells to expand or increase in size. It is the fluid replacement of choice for diarrhea and dehydration.

> *Nursing Process:* Implementation
> *Client Needs:* Physiological Integrity
> *Clinical Area:* Pediatric Nursing

69. (2) Semi-Fowler's position—in an infant seat—is the position of choice, because it allows for lung expansion that facilitates breathing.

> *Nursing Process:* Implementation
> *Client Needs:* Safe, Effective Care Environment
> *Clinical Area:* Pediatric Nursing

70. (1) Clients taking phenothiazines are sensitive to the sun (photophobia). The correct answer is to have these clients put on sunscreen and wear hats when they are in the sun. Answer (4) refers to an MAO inhibiting drug used for depression.

> *Nursing Process:* Implementation
> *Client Needs:* Safe, Effective Care Environment
> *Clinical Area:* Psychiatric Nursing

71. (3) Diabetes insipidus results from a condition related to hypofunction of the posterior pituitary gland. Clients experience severe polyuria and eliminate large volumes of fluid resulting in a dehydration state. Urine output and specific gravity values assist with assessing fluid balance.

> *Nursing Process:* Data Collection
> *Client Needs:* Physiological Integrity
> *Clinical Area:* Medical Nursing

72. (3) Proper alignment is critical to maintain skeletal traction in counterbalance or correct pull. It is also important to assess for pressure points or skin excoriation, but these observations would be continual as long as the traction is in place.

> *Nursing Process:* Data Collection
> *Client Needs:* Safe, Effective Care Environment
> *Clinical Area:* Surgical Nursing

73. (1) If physiological jaundice goes above 13 mg/100 mL of blood, phototherapy is ordered. The protocol of this therapy—fluorescent lights to break down bilirubin into water soluble products—is to keep the infant uncovered and to cover the infant's eyes to prevent retinal damage. This is not an infection, so answer (3) is incorrect, and the nurse would not avoid handling the infant. In fact, the nurse would change the newborn's position every 2 hours and cuddle for feedings.

> *Nursing Process:* Implementation
> *Client Needs:* Safe, Effective Care Environment
> *Clinical Area:* Maternity Nursing

74. (2) The most important nursing care directed toward preventing ulcer extension or development is to reposition the client—turn her from side-to-side—at least every 2 hours.

> *Nursing Process:* Planning
> *Client Needs:* Safe, Effective Care Environment
> *Clinical Area:* Medical Nursing

75. (2) The most specific reason for applying a wet-to-dry dressing and wringing out excess moisture is to leave only enough moisture to dry between dressing changes. The dead material is trapped in the dressing, and when it is removed, the necrotic material is also removed. Answer (3) is not as direct and specific an answer.

> *Nursing Process:* Planning
> *Client Needs:* Safe, Effective Care Environment
> *Clinical Area:* Medical Nursing

76. (4) A severe allergic reaction requires that the nurse stop the transfusion immediately. The second action is to check for a patent airway. The nurse would then notify the physician.

> *Nursing Process:* Implementation
> *Client Needs:* Safe, Effective Care Environment
> *Clinical Area:* Medical Nursing

77. (3) The primary side effects of the drug, Dilantin, are bleeding gums and gum hypertrophy, rash and GI symptoms. Answer (3) is the preferable choice because it will involve teaching the client to use a soft toothbrush, brush frequently, and eat a diet high in vitamins and minerals to protect the gums. Dilantin does not cause mood disturbances, drowsiness or ataxia.

> *Nursing Process:* Implementation
> *Client Needs:* Health Promotion and Maintenance
> *Clinical Area:* Pediatric Nursing

78. (4) It is important that the client not bear weight on the affected hip. She is likely to be ambulated directly from her bed to a walker on the second postoperative day. The nursing responsibility is to ensure that the client avoid positions with 60 to 90 degree angles, such as sitting on the side of the bed or in a chair.

> *Nursing Process:* Implementation
> *Client Needs:* Health Promotion and Maintenance
> *Clinical Area:* Surgical Nursing

79. (1) Once a decision is made to commit suicide, the client often feels relieved and presents an attitude and demeanor of calmness and satisfaction. The client may even state that "everything is falling into place" or "now, everything will be all right." When a client is in a deep depression, he does not have the energy to formulate or follow through on a suicide plan. Expressing anger may be interpreted as a positive sign, because the anger is directed outward, not inward. Answer (3) may also be a positive sign of improvement.

Nursing Process: Evaluation
Client Needs: Psychosocial Integrity
Clinical Area: Psychiatric Nursing

80. (2) One of the goals of therapy is to build the client's self-esteem. Helping another client may accomplish this goal. Answer (1) is not appropriate, because the client may not be ready for group therapy. Answer (3) will not do much to raise her self-esteem. Because this client finds it difficult to focus and concentrate, learning to knit may not be therapeutic, but stressful.

Nursing Process: Implementation
Client Needs: Psychosocial Integrity
Clinical Area: Psychiatric Nursing

81. (4) The issue in this question is safety; therefore, the most important nursing action is to check that the number on the record and the blood bag match. The nurse will check for all of the essential data: client's name, ID number, blood group and type, blood unit number, and expiration date of the blood. All of the other answers are appropriate to carry out, but the issue is safety.

Nursing Process: Planning
Client Needs: Safe, Effective Care Environment
Clinical Area: Medical Nursing

82. (1) A side effect of atropine sulfate is a dry mouth. Telling the client he can expect to experience this side effect will help to decrease the anxiety which he may be feeling due to his scheduled surgery.

Nursing Process: Evaluation
Client Needs: Health Promotion and Maintenance
Clinical Area: Medical Nursing

83. (3) Suctioning longer than this length of time will remove excess oxygen and this may lead to hypoxemia. Another technique of preventing hypoxemia is to administer oxygen 1 to 2 minutes before suctioning.

Nursing Process: Implementation
Client Needs: Safe, Effective Care Environment
Clinical Area: Surgical Nursing

84. (3) Vitamin B_{12} will have to be replaced for the remainder of the client's life because gastric secretion is required for the absorption of B_{12}. The gastric surgery resulted in the absence of the "intrinsic factor." Unless Vitamin B_{12} is supplied by parenteral injection, the client will experience a deficiency of this nutrient.

Nursing Process: Implementation
Client Needs: Health Promotion and Maintenance
Clinical Area: Surgical Nursing

85. (3) Credé is a French term that refers to the manual expression of urine, made necessary because of a hypotonic bladder. This method will help initiate bladder retraining.

Nursing Process: Planning
Client Needs: Safe, Effective Care Environment
Clinical Area: Medical Nursing

86. (2) The end of the drainage tube is kept under water; this water seals the tube so air cannot enter and be drawn back into the pleural space.

Nursing Process: Planning
Client Needs: Safe, Effective Care Environment
Clinical Area: Medical Nursing

87. (1) Prevention of thrombophlebitis involves several nursing actions; one of the most important is to encourage feet and leg exercises, 10 minutes every 2 hours. The nurse would

NOT massage the calf, gatch the bed, or place pillows under the knees, because all of these measures would contribute to the development of thrombophlebitis.

Nursing Process: Implementation
Client Needs: Safe, Effective Care Environment
Clinical Area: Surgical Nursing

88. (3) The IV calorie calculation formula is as follows:

° 1000 mL D_5W provides 50 gm of dextrose.
° 50 gm of dextrose provides four calories per gram; thus, multiply 50 gm x 4 calories.
° 1000 mL D_5W provides 200 calories.
° Usual IV total per day is 3000 mL or 600 calories per day.

Nursing Process: Planning
Client Needs: Safe, Effective Care Environment
Clinical Area: Medical Nursing

89. (2) The possibility exists that the client could hemorrhage from the stump. Therefore, it is safe nursing care to have a tourniquet at the bedside. The dressing is not changed unless ordered, and the prone position is usually not indicated until the first postoperative day.

Nursing Process: Implementation
Client Needs: Safe, Effective Care Environment
Clinical Area: Surgical Nursing

90. (2) A diet with restricted potassium and protein is necessary for all children who demonstrate some degree of renal failure.

Nursing Process: Implementation
Client Needs: Physiological Integrity
Clinical Area: Pediatric Nursing

COMPREHENSIVE TEST 2

1. A male client has been given the diagnosis hepatitis B. When the nurse is assessing his understanding of the disease, he tells her that the nursing assistant told him the only precaution necessary is for him to wash his hands. The appropriate nursing action is to

   1 Confront the nursing assistant about the information she told the client.
   2 Teach the client how to correctly wash his hands.
   3 Teach both client and nursing assistant additional precautions.
   4 Validate for the client that the statement is true.

2. A child is admitted to the hospital with marked symptoms of nephrosis. The following information should be included in the admission nurse's notes. Which information is *most pertinent* in terms of the child's condition?

   1 Color of the skin and mucous membranes.
   2 Pattern of bowel elimination and extent of bowel training.
   3 Degree and distribution of edema.
   4 Pulse and respiratory rate and temperature.

3. In an Rh negative female, the *most common* cause of sensitization to the Rh factor is

   1 Deficiency of immunoglobulins.
   2 Pregnancy with an Rh positive baby.
   3 Transfusion with improperly matched blood types.
   4 Pregnancy with an Rh negative baby.

4. A new mother tells the nurse that she wishes to breast feed. The postpartum nurse should begin her teaching with

   1 Anatomy and physiology of breast feeding.

   2 An assessment of the mother's knowledge base.
   3 A dietary assessment and nutrition counseling.
   4 Instructions on breast feeding techniques.

5. A client comes to the clinic for a follow-up visit after a severe angina attack. The nurse asks him if he continues to experience symptoms. He states that he has some pain but "it's probably from something I ate." This reaction can best be explained by the statement that the client

   1 Is probably developing a stress ulcer.
   2 Is probably eating spicy foods and developing gastritis.
   3 Does not know how angina feels and must be taught.
   4 May be having angina pain but is denying it.

6. A 42-year-old female client is brought to the hospital by her daughter. The admitting diagnosis is depressive episode. She says there is nothing to live for since her husband died and her future is hopeless. The nurse can best respond to this communication by saying

   1 "You don't want to talk like that. It will only depress you more."
   2 "Let's talk about when you were growing up. You mentioned that you had lived in Vermont."
   3 "Tell me more about feeling hopeless and worthless."
   4 "Talking about these things seems to make you feel worse. Let's go to the activity room and you and I can join the exercise group."

7. A 60-year-old female client has a tentative diagnosis of myocardial infarction (MI). Which

one of the following laboratory values is the *best* indicator of an MI?

1 CPK-MB.
2 LDH1.
3 SGOT.
4 WBC.

8. The instructions to a client just learning to use a four-point crutch-walking gait would be to move the

1 Right foot, then the right crutch.
2 Right crutch, then the right foot.
3 Right crutch, then the left foot.
4 Left foot, then the left crutch.

9. An 8-year-old male child is admitted to the hospital during an acute asthma attack. Epinephrine has just been administered by inhalation. Oxygen is ordered PRN. The child becomes short of breath with circumoral cyanosis and sweating. The appropriate nursing action is to

1 Notify the physician immediately.
2 Encourage the child to lie down and administer oxygen.
3 Reassure the child that the medication will begin working soon.
4 Encourage the child to sit upright and administer oxygen.

10. A 55-year-old female client has been on bedrest for 2 days following surgery and the nurse is completing a general assessment of her condition. Which of the following is an *initial* sign of thrombophlebitis?

1 A positive Homan's sign.
2 Calf pain and edema.
3 Difficulty breathing.
4 Distended vein collaterals.

11. A 1-month-old female infant has been readmitted to the hospital for a cleft lip repair. In

planning for her preoperative care, the nurse will feed her in a/an

1 Upright position with a regular nipple.
2 Side-lying position with a soft nipple.
3 Infant seat in slant position with a medicine dropper.
4 Upright position with a cross-cut nipple.

12. A male client has been diagnosed with Pneumocystis carinii. Caring for this client, the nurse would be most in danger of contracting AIDS while

1 Starting an IV.
2 Spiking a blood bag.
3 Taping an IV site.
4 Performing naso-oral suctioning.

13. When caring for a 5-month-old child in the hospital, the *best* toy or object for stimulation would be a

1 Hanging mobile.
2 Teddy bear.
3 Toy that makes noise.
4 Fabric picture book.

14. An adult male client is admitted to the hospital for a cardiac work-up. During the initial physical assessment, the nurse listens for bronchovesicular breath sounds. These sounds can normally be heard over the

1 Lung base.
2 Trachea above the sternal notch.
3 Mainstem bronchi below the clavicle.
4 Entire lung parenchyma.

15. A young client, age 12, is hospitalized for left lower lobe pneumonia. The physician has ordered percussion, vibration and postural drainage for as long as tolerated or 30 minutes. Prior to providing this intervention, the nursing priority action is to

1 Give instructions on correct diaphragmatic breathing.

2   Assess vital signs.
3   Auscultate lung fields.
4   Assess sputum characteristics.

16. A male client has a tracheostomy and requires suctioning. The nurse knows that signs of hypoxia may occur during this procedure. A nursing action to prevent hypoxia is to

1   Ensure that the catheter is no more than three-quarters the diameter of the tube.
2   Limit suction time to 30 seconds at intervals of 3 minutes.
3   Hyperinflate the lungs with 100% oxygen prior to and following suctioning.
4   Suction no more than three consecutive times before administering oxygen.

17. A male client has had a lobectomy for cancer of the left lower lobe of the lung. Eighteen hours following surgery, the most appropriate position for this client is

1   Flat bedrest.
2   Turned to the unoperative side only.
3   Turned to the operative side only.
4   Semi-Fowler's position, turned to either side.

18. To ensure a smooth transition from hospital to home, the nurse's discharge planning would depend most on

1   Discharge from the hospital when the client is independent.
2   Adequate physician instructions to the family.
3   An appropriate and complete discharge plan prior to discharge.
4   Complete client teaching while in the hospital.

19. A 24-year-old married female suspects that she is pregnant. She states that her last menstrual period started on August 9, 1996. She asks, "If I am pregnant, when will my baby be due?" According to Nägele's rule, the due date would be

1   May 16, 1997.
2   April 13, 1997.
3   January 12, 1997.
4   June 6, 1997.

20. A female client has the diagnosis of cerebral vascular accident (CVA) and has been in the hospital for 3 days. Physician's orders include oxygen 6 L/minute, elevate head of bed and supportive care. Considering the physician's orders, the nurse will instruct the nursing assistant to carry out a positioning schedule of

1   Changing her position every 2 hours.
2   Maintaining elevation of the head of the bed at 20 degrees and changing position every 2 hours.
3   Keeping her in high-Fowler's position and changing her from unaffected to affected side every 2 hours.
4   Keeping her very quiet, but rotating positions every 4 hours.

21. A 1½-year-old is brought to the hospital with a diagnosis of pneumonia. His temperature is 38.8° C (102° F), respiratory rate is 40 and he appears lethargic. A tentative diagnosis of pneumonia is made. Evaluating his condition, an indication that he is improving is a respiratory rate of

1   30 per minute.
2   18 per minute.
3   20 per minute.
4   50 per minute.

22. A new mother-to-be asks why her doctor told her to discontinue taking all unnecessary drugs during pregnancy. Based on the understanding of the relationship between drugs and the fetus, the nurse's reply would be

1   "Your doctor is just being safe. There is some research to support the belief that common drugs affect the fetus."
2   "Some drugs can cause deformity, but most do not pass through the placental barrier to the fetus."

3 "All drugs can cross the placental barrier and may be dangerous."

4 "Drugs should be avoided in pregnancy, especially during the last trimester."

23. Adequate nutrition is essential during early pregnancy for optimum fetal development. The nurse recommends a daily diet that would include

1 Low roughage foods.
2 One fruit or vegetable high in vitamin C.
3 A low-sodium diet.
4 1500 calories.

24. A 28-year-old male client with a suspected brain tumor is admitted to the hospital. While assessing this client, the nurse keeps in mind that the most reliable index of neurological status is

1 Pupil response.
2 Deep tendon reflexes.
3 Muscle strength.
4 Level of consciousness.

25. When the nurse assesses the condition of a client with a suspected brain tumor, she observes that his intracranial pressure has increased. The nursing intervention is to

1 Chart the increase on the client's chart.
2 Report the increase at the change of shift.
3 Report the increase to the charge nurse immediately.
4 Do nothing, because this change is to be expected.

26. A cerebral arteriogram is performed on the client. When he returns from the operating room, the nurse observes that he may be having a reaction to the dye. The sign or symptom that suggests this complication is

1 A severe headache.
2 Numbness of the extremities.

3 Hypertension.
4 Polyuria.

27. The client goal for fluid intake following abdominal surgery for an inguinal hernia would be

1 500 to 700 mL/day.
2 1000 to 1500 mL/day.
3 2000 to 3000 mL/day. ✓
4 3000 to 3500 mL/day.

28. The nursing assistant informs the nurse that the client's IV is running fast and he has received 1000 mL in less than an hour. When checking his condition, the nurse would expect to observe

1 Hyperventilation.
2 Dyspnea.
3 Bradycardia.
4 Hypertension.

29. A 26-year-old primigravida is mildly preeclamptic and will be followed on an outpatient basis. Which of the following signs or symptoms should the nurse expect to observe if the eclampsia is becoming more severe?

1 Edema of the hands, feet and face.
2 Glycosuria.
3 Hypotension.
4 Polyuria.

30. Case finding and evaluation are very important for good prenatal care. The conditions *most often* related to diabetic pregnancies are

1 Abruptio placenta, eclampsia, obesity.
2 Familial diabetes, unexplained stillbirths, obesity.
3 Habitual abortion, placenta previa, malnutrition.
4 Hydatidiform mole, excessive sized infants, twin gestation.

31. The RN has discussed the baby's newborn status with the mother and asks the practical nurse to reinforce it. She explains to the mother that the insulin level in newborns of diabetic mothers

  1 Is higher than in normal infants.
  2 Is lower than in normal infants.
  3 Is the same as in normal infants.
  4 Varies from baby to baby.

32. The client has a diagnosis of acute depression. As the nurse goes into her room, she is crying and says, "I've screwed everything up. It's hopeless. It's no use." The *most appropriate* response to these feelings of hopelessness is

  1 "You've screwed everything up?"
  2 "Why do you feel it's no use?"
  3 "Sometimes we have to hit bottom before things get better."
  4 "You sound like you're feeling very despondent. Are you thinking about harming yourself?"

33. A client who has been depressed, noncommunicative, and unable to join in activities begins to participate in her treatment program. An indication that the client is ready for discharge will be when she

  1 Has formulated a plan to return home and continue therapy.
  2 Has talked to her boss about returning to work.
  3 Has identified her weak areas and is working on them.
  4 Is now asking the staff for advice about her future.

34. A client is admitted to the hospital with leg ulcers, venous insufficiency and a diagnosis of Raynaud's disease. The nursing care plan for this client will include interventions that focus on

  1 Buerger-Allen exercises.
  2 Exercises to increase collateral circulation.

  3 Thigh high TEDs at all times.
  4 Antigravity measures.

35. A client is being prepared for an oral cholecystogram. Before the dinner meal the practical nurse instructs the nursing assistant to

  1 Provide a regular diet for dinner, then NPO.
  2 Give the client tea and toast and explain that diarrhea may result from the dye tablets.
  3 Administer the dye tablets with a regular dinner.
  4 Administer enemas until clear after a regular meal.

36. A 7-year-old male complains of pain and limited movement in his left hip. The physician suspects Legg-Perthes disease. At this stage of the disease, the major goal of treatment is aimed at

  1 Preventing deformity in the shaft of the femur.
  2 Preventing degenerative changes in the knee joint.
  3 Reducing muscle spasm.
  4 Preventing pressure on the head of the femur.

37. The client is age 4 and while in the hospital, he becomes very bored. The *best* activity to implement for this client is

  1 Radio and TV.
  2 Puppets.
  3 Books and comics.
  4 Airplane models.

38. A 34-year-old male client with a diagnosis of schizophrenia, paranoid type, barges into the dayroom yelling, "The President is on my side. If you bother me, I'll send him after you!" The nurse could *most effectively* respond by saying

1 "We do not allow threatening behavior here."
2 "You don't expect me to believe the President is a friend of yours!"
3 "I understand you are concerned. The staff will see that you are safe."
4 "What do you think we're going to do to bother you?"

39. A male client was admitted with a diagnosis of subdural hematoma and transferred to the ICU in a semicomatose state. If the client goes into a coma, the nurse would be likely to observe

1 Decreased blood pressure, tachypnea.
2 Decreased blood pressure, bradycardia.
3 Increased blood pressure, bradypnea.
4 Increased blood pressure, tachycardia.

40. A male client is taken to surgery for evacuation of a subdural hematoma. Immediately after the evacuation, the *priority* nursing assessment is to observe

1 For CSF leaks around the evacuation site.
2 Temperature for signs of infection.
3 That airway remains patent.
4 For signs of increasing intracranial pressure.

41. The physician has ordered electroconvulsive therapy (ECT) for a 65-year-old client. ECT is considered *most effective* in treating elderly clients with symptoms of

1 Phobic reactions.
2 Depression.
3 Schizophrenia.
4 Paranoid reactions.

42. Which of the following is the *most common* side effect of electroconvulsive therapy (ECT)?

1 Loss of memory.
2 Nausea and vomiting.
3 Constipation.
4 Loss of balance.

43. A female client has sustained burns of her right arm, right chest, face, and neck. She has just been admitted to the burn unit. Her weight on admission is 50 kg. Using the rule of nines, the estimate of the extent of her burns is

1 27 percent.
2 22.5 percent.
3 36 percent.
4 15 percent.

44. To promote adequate nutrition, a burn client's diet after the first week of hospitalization should include

1 High protein, low sodium, low carbohydrate.
2 Low fat, low sodium, high calorie.
3 High protein, high carbohydrate.
4 High protein, high vitamin B complex, low sodium.

45. A teenager has just been told she has herpes simplex II. When discussing the test results with her, she says, "That's not possible. I've only slept with my boyfriend." The *best* response would be

1 "Well, then, he has probably slept with someone else who infected him."
2 "It's all right to tell me the truth. Our conversation is confidential."
3 "Can you tell me what you know about herpes?"
4 "How you got it doesn't really matter. What's important is that we treat it now."

46. Discussing nutrition with a pregnant teenager, the nurse helps her select the *best* protein source from the choices in the school cafeteria by suggesting that she choose

1 A slice of pizza.
2 Macaroni.
3 A peanut butter sandwich.
4 Tomato soup.

47. Each newborn receives an Apgar score shortly after birth. The nurse understands that the purpose of Apgar scoring is to

    1 Determine the viability status.
    2 Assess for congenital anomalies.
    3 Assess the cardiac and respiratory status.
    4 Evaluate the Rh status.

48. The physician orders that a newborn be placed in a heated isolette in Trendelenburg position. The rationale for this therapy is to

    1 Prevent loss of heat and facilitate drainage of mucus.
    2 Increase oxygen intake.
    3 Allow more blood to flow to the brain.
    4 Provide an environment similar to the uterus.

49. Included in the nursing care plan is the goal of monitoring the humidity in the isolette. The purpose of humidifying the air is to

    1 Improve cardiac rhythm.
    2 Prevent hyperbilirubinemia.
    3 Increase the infant's temperature.
    4 Prevent drying of bronchial secretions.

50. The nurse recognizes that it is important to monitor the O_2 concentration that a newborn receives, because high levels of oxygen may cause

    1 Kernicterus.
    2 Blindness.
    3 Peripheral circulatory collapse.
    4 Respiratory complications.

51. The nurse is counseling a male client whose discharge orders include nitroglycerin. Teaching instructions will include that if the client receives no relief after 15 minutes with 2 tablets, he should

    1 Take a third tablet and wait another 15 minutes.
    2 Notify his physician immediately.

    3 Relax and deep breathe for the next 15 minutes.
    4 Call his physician and request a change in medication.

52. A 20-year-old male client, after experiencing thyroid dysfunction due to a tumor, is admitted to the hospital for a subtotal thyroidectomy. Immediate postoperative care includes correct positioning. The appropriate position is

    1 Semi-Fowler's with neck erect.
    2 High-Fowler's with neck extended.
    3 Semi-Fowler's with neck flexed.
    4 Sims' with neck extended.

53. The nurse has completed a postoperative assessment for hypoparathyroidism following a thyroidectomy. If the symptoms of this condition are present, the nurse would check with the RN and expect to administer

    1 Calcium gluconate.
    2 Magnesium sulfate.
    3 Diazepam (Valium).
    4 Anectine.

54. A client is admitted to the hospital with an obstruction just proximal to the old ileostomy stoma. The nurse will monitor for a major complication which is most likely to be

    1 Infection.
    2 Diarrhea.
    3 Fluid and electrolyte imbalance.
    4 Constipation.

55. The nurse will know that a client with an ileostomy understands dietary restrictions when she indicates that she does not include which one of the following foods in her diet?

    1 Cabbage.
    2 Corn.
    3 Red meat.
    4 Radishes.

56. A young male client was admitted with symptoms of hypertension, edema, headache, and oliguria. The diagnosis of glomerulonephritis was made. When he suddenly starts complaining of a severe headache, the nurse's *first* intervention is to

 1 Call the physician.
 2 Raise him to a Fowler's position.
 3 Take his blood pressure.
 4 Administer a PRN pain medication.

57. The physician has just completed a liver biopsy on an elderly female client. Immediately following the procedure, the nurse will position the client

 1 On her right side to promote hemostasis.
 2 In Fowler's position to facilitate ventilation.
 3 Supine to maintain blood pressure.
 4 In Sims' position to prevent aspiration.

58. A 54-year-old male client with a history of cirrhosis from alcohol abuse has been admitted for bleeding esophageal varices. While the client is on bedrest, he is in a semi-Fowler's position. The major objective for using this position is to

 1 Lower portal pressure.
 2 Allow for effective breathing.
 3 Decrease blood pressure.
 4 Decrease risk of aspiration from vomiting.

59. The nurse is assisting the physician to insert a Sengstaken-Blakemore tube. Prior to insertion the nursing action is to

 1 Insert mercury into the gastric balloon.
 2 Clamp the NG suction lumen.
 3 Check both balloons for leaks.
 4 Insert mercury into the esophageal balloon.

60. A child with the diagnosis of phenylketonuria (PKU) may not eat which of the following foods?

 1 Chocolate.
 2 Lima beans.
 3 Carrots.
 4 Applesauce.

61. After cataract surgery, a client tells the nurse she is worried about a cataract forming in the other eye and asks how she will know if this is happening. The nurse should teach the client by responding

 1 "You will see a white halo when you look at lights."
 2 "You will see floating spots before your eyes."
 3 "You will notice blurred vision."
 4 "You will have difficulty seeing at night."

62. A male client has advanced cirrhosis. His blood test results have been returned and indicate a prothrombin time of 30 seconds. The nurse would expect the physician to order

 1 Vitamin K.
 2 Heparin.
 3 Coumadin.
 4 Ferrous sulfate.

63. When a client with advanced cirrhosis selects a snack, the choice that indicates understanding of the dietary requirements is

 1 A peanut butter sandwich.
 2 One banana.
 3 A hard boiled egg.
 4 Cheese and crackers.

64. A 74-year-old male client with a diagnosis of senile dementia is in a long-term care facility. Late one night the nurse finds him wandering around the halls. He says he is looking for his wife. The most therapeutic approach is to

1 Use a matter-of-fact attitude and help him back to his room.
2 Remind him he should stay in his room.
3 Remind him of where he is and assess why he is having difficulty sleeping.
4 Allow him to sleep in the dayroom so he will not disturb the other clients.

65. A 12-year-old client with a tentative diagnosis of diabetes mellitus asks the nurse for a dish of ice cream. Which of the following responses by the nurse would be *best*?

1 "You know diabetics can't have ice cream. It has too much sugar."
2 "You'll have to check with the dietitian."
3 "Okay, I'll get you some and check your blood sugar in 1 hour."
4 "You'll have to give up 1 glass of milk and 2 teaspoons of butter."

66. Which of the following assessments of the client with an abdominal aortic aneurysm requires immediate reporting to the physician?

1 Blood pressure increasing from 120/80 to 160/90.
2 Bruit heard over an abdominal mass.
3 Palpation of a pulsating mass left of the midline.
4 Client verbalizes some anxiety about the upcoming surgical procedure.

67. A client is having a prolonged labor and there is no progress past a dilation of 8 cm. Her physician decides to do a cesarean delivery. The new mother and her partner express their disappointment that they will not have a natural childbirth. The *best* response is to say

1 "Most couples who have an unplanned cesarean birth feel cheated and disappointed."
2 "You know that at least you will have a healthy baby."
3 "Maybe next time you can have a vaginal delivery."
4 "You will be able to resume sex sooner than if you have a vaginal delivery."

68. The nurse assigned to care for a newborn understands that the purpose of instilling a broad spectrum antibiotic or silver nitrate in the newborn infant's eyes is to prevent

1 Erythroblastosis fetalis.
2 Retrolental fibroplasia.
3 Ophthalmia neonatorum.
4 Icterus neonatorum.

69. The nursing goal that is *most important* to include in a care plan for a client with congestive heart failure is to

1 Allow the client to exercise and be out of bed ad lib.
2 Maintain alternate rest and exercise periods for the client.
3 Provide the client with frequent exercise periods.
4 Maintain the client on bedrest at all times.

70. A 1-year-old child is admitted to the hospital with a diagnosis of bronchiolitis. Collecting data on her condition, the nurse will observe for

1 Retractions and inspiratory stridor.
2 Flaring of nostrils and expiratory stridor with wheezing and grunting.
3 Rapid, shallow respirations accompanied by severe, subcostal retractions.
4 Elevated temperature and expiratory stridor.

71. A client with a diagnosis of compulsive disorder often arrives late to meals and does not have time to finish eating because of her schedule of pacing before any activity. The appropriate nursing action is to

1 Plan to provide her meals later and after the others have eaten.
2 Notify her 30 minutes before the meal so she can complete her pacing before eating.
3 Interrupt the pacing and insist she come to meals with everyone else.
4 Allow her to continue as is, but provide her access to the kitchen.

72. A client with the diagnosis of ritualistic behavior is scheduled for group therapy. The nurse will plan that this activity occur

   1 Before the client begins her ritual in the morning and becomes too anxious.
   2 In the middle of the ritual, because this is the optimal time for a low anxiety level.
   3 In the evening, when the client's anxiety is low after having performed the ritual all day.
   4 After the client has just completed the ritual.

73. The team leader overhears a new LVN graduate assigning the nursing assistant (NA) to check on a client who has just returned from surgery following a transurethral prostatic resection (TURP). He has a 3-way Foley catheter inserted. The LVN has asked the NA to see if the catheter is draining. The team leader's intervention would be to

   1 Remind the LVN to chart the drainage from the catheter because the physician will want to know.
   2 Do nothing because this assignment is appropriate for the NA.
   3 Instruct the LVN that this is not an appropriate assignment for the NA.
   4 Tell the new graduate that she will check on the client herself and report back to the charge nurse.

74. A 20-year-old female client is admitted in a comatose state to the emergency room. Her vital signs are BP 140/80, P 110, R 30 and labored. A MedicAlert bracelet indicates that she is a diabetic. If the nurse were assessing her for ketoacidosis, one significant symptom would be

   1 Oliguria.
   2 Acetone odor to breath.
   3 Kussmaul breathing.
   4 Sensorium change.

75. A 58-year-old client is in the hospital recovering from a CVA. The physician has ordered a mineral oil disposable enema. The position the nurse will place her in before administering the enema is

   1 Left side in prone position.
   2 Left side in Sims' position.
   3 Right side in side-lying position.
   4 Semi-Fowler's with knees up.

76. At which of the following ages would the nurse first expect a child to sit with no support?

   1 Four months.
   2 Five months.
   3 Eight months.
   4 Nine months.

77. The parents of a 4 month old noticed that many bruises were forming on their son's knees, buttocks and thighs. The blood tests reveal that he has classic hemophilia. The nurse understands that hemophilia is

   1 Caused by spontaneous mutation.
   2 Transmitted by diseased mothers to affected sons on the X chromosome.
   3 Transmitted by asymptomatic fathers to affected sons on the Y chromosome.
   4 Transmitted by asymptomatic females to affected sons on the X chromosome.

78. A 4-month-old infant has been spitting up his feedings and the mother asks for advice. What instructions will the nurse give to the mother?

   1 Carefully feed him the correct amount of formula for his age.
   2 Reduce the amount of formula given at one time.
   3 Feed him slowly with a small-holed nipple.
   4 Change him before feeding, but not after.

79. The *initial* treatment of children with rheumatic fever consists of the administration of drugs such as

    1 Penicillin and salicylates.
    2 Antihypertensives.
    3 Aspirin and digitalis.
    4 Phenobarbital or morphine.

80. The public health department is responsible for providing an immunization program in this country. In planning the program, their primary aim is to

    1 Have every child immunized.
    2 Immunize 80 percent of the child population.
    3 Immunize 60 percent of the child population.
    4 Have each community make decisions on immunization based on its own needs.

81. While on the unit one day, the nurse observes an RN unlock the narcotic cabinet, look around, then put a vial of morphine sulfate in her pocket. The appropriate action under these circumstances would be to

    1 Ignore the behavior this time, but "keep your eye" on the nurse.
    2 Confront the nurse and ask her why she is doing it.
    3 Report observations to the charge nurse.
    4 Call the police, because taking narcotics is illegal.

82. A drug commonly administered to reduce the extrapyramidal side effects of phenothiazines used in the treatment of schizophrenia is

    1 Cogentin.
    2 Niamid.
    3 Ritalin.
    4 Valium.

83. A 2 year old has eaten half a bottle of his grandmother's ferrous sulfate tablets. When the mother calls in, the nurse will tell the mother to

    1 Take him to the hospital immediately.
    2 Give him syrup of ipecac to induce vomiting.
    3 Contact the poison control center by phone.
    4 Do nothing because vitamins are nonpoisonous.

84. A 58-year-old client with a diagnosis of schizophrenia, chronic undifferentiated type is taking 400 mg of chlorpromazine (Thorazine) TID. The nurse notices on the morning rounds that he is drooling and flapping when he walks. The *best* nursing action would be to

    1 Provide activities away from other clients so he will not be embarrassed.
    2 Call the physician immediately about the toxic effects of the drug.
    3 Chart and discuss observations with the charge nurse so that a medication to control these symptoms can be ordered.
    4 Hold his next dose of Thorazine.

85. A 65-year-old female client has suffered a cerebral vascular accident (CVA)—left hemisphere lesion. The *most appropriate* method of communicating with her is to

    1 Speak in a loud voice so that she can understand what is being said.
    2 Draw pictures, because the client cannot understand words.
    3 Act out or pantomime communication while speaking in a normal tone of voice.
    4 Use only verbal cues as demonstrations, because pantomime will confuse the client.

86. The client has a diagnosis of gall bladder disease. When he is admitted, his oral temperature is 38.3° C (101° F) and the lab reports a white blood cell count of 15,000 per cu mm. The *most appropriate* nursing intervention is to

1 Observe for signs of dehydration that will increase with a high temperature.
2 Notify the physician immediately, because this is not an expected clinical picture.
3 Follow admission orders, because these findings are to be expected.
4 Increase the IV as ordered, because these clinical manifestations indicate an increased need for fluid.

87. A young client, following a motorcycle accident, sustained spinal cord injury with respiratory function impairment. The cord segments involved with maintaining respiratory function are

1 Thoracic level 5 and 6.
2 Thoracic level 2 and 3.
3 Cervical level 7 and 8.
4 Cervical level 3 and 4.

88. The nurse is assigned a client with the diagnosis of portal hypertension. The *most important* assessment with this condition is for the complication of

1 Jaundice.
2 Weight gain.
3 Low urine output.
4 GI bleeding.

89. An elderly client with organic brain syndrome suffers from insomnia and asks the nurse for something to help him sleep. The physician will *not* order barbiturates for this client because they cause

1 Potential liver damage.
2 Habituation and dependence.
3 Delirium and paradoxical excitement.
4 Central nervous system depression.

90. A diabetic client takes 22 units of NPH insulin at 7:30 AM each day. Evaluating the effects of insulin, at which time during the day will the nurse assess her for signs of restlessness, memory lapses and headache?

1 8:30 AM.
2 10:30 AM.
3 3:30 PM.
4 5:00 AM.

COMPREHENSIVE TEST 2

Answers with Rationale

1. (3) Both the client and nursing assistant need the correct information and to be taught that the oral, parenteral or sexual route can be modes of transmission. Good handwashing is important to prevent transmission of hepatitis A.

    Nursing Process: Data Collection
    Client Needs: Safe, Effective Care Environment
    Clinical Area: Medical Nursing

2. (3) It is important to note the degree and extent of generalized edema that occurs with nephrosis. The condition is characterized by severe proteinuria which results in hypoalbuminuria leading to the shift of fluid from the intravascular to the extracellular compartment.

    Nursing Process: Data Collection
    Client Needs: Physiological Integrity
    Clinical Area: Pediatric Nursing

3. (2) An Rh negative mother will become sensitized to the Rh factor by carrying an Rh positive baby. If she is pregnant with a second Rh positive baby, it could result in erythroblastosis. This condition is now rare due to the use of RhoGAM.

    Nursing Process: Planning
    Client Needs: Physiological Integrity
    Clinical Area: Maternity Nursing

4. (2) The principles of client teaching always begin with assessing the client's knowledge base and making a plan based on the preexisting knowledge.

    Nursing Process: Evaluation
    Client Needs: Health Promotion and Maintenance
    Clinical Area: Maternity Nursing

5. (4) This client seems to be in denial and unable to face the reality of his condition. The ego protects itself from conflict by rejecting reality, and denial of illness is a common example.

    Nursing Process: Evaluation
    Client Needs: Psychosocial Integrity
    Clinical Area: Medical Nursing

6. (4) The most therapeutic response is to acknowledge the communication and, at the same time, assist the client to mobilize, do an activity, and focus on something other than depressed thoughts. (1) This response is maternal and nontherapeutic. Also, it does not acknowledge the client's feelings. (2) The nurse has changed the subject to a tangential topic. This form of response is nontherapeutic, because it cuts off the client and does not acknowledge her communication. (3) Exploring the feelings, when they center around hopelessness and self-denigration, is nontherapeutic; focusing on them will only increase the depression.

    Nursing Process: Implementation
    Client Needs: Psychosocial Integrity
    Clinical Area: Psychiatric Nursing

7. (1) All of these laboratory studies provide information about the condition, but the CPK-MB is the most valuable measurement. The level rises within 6 hours of myocardial cell death and remains elevated for about 3 days.

Nursing Process: Planning
Client Needs: Physiological Integrity
Clinical Area: Medical Nursing

8. (3) The crutch is always moved first, and then the foot on the opposite side is moved forward.

Nursing Process: Implementation
Client Needs: Safe, Effective Care Environment
Clinical Area: Medical Nursing

9. (4) The correct nursing action to promote respiratory exchange is to sit the child up and administer oxygen. Epinephrine will begin to work to reduce congestion and edema so answer (3) is a subsequent intervention that will help to reduce anxiety.

Nursing Process: Implementation
Client Needs: Safe, Effective Care Environment
Clinical Area: Pediatric Nursing

10. (2) Edema and pain in the affected leg usually appear first, accompanied by warm skin. Chills and fever may also be present. Pulmonary embolism frequently occurs as the first indication of a clot in over half of the clients with venous thrombosis. In this case, dyspnea and pain would be present.

Nursing Process: Data Collection
Client Needs: Physiological Integrity
Clinical Area: Medical Nursing

11. (4) An upright or sitting position is important when using a soft, large-holed, cross-cut or special nipple. The nipple should be placed on the opposite side from the cleft.

Nursing Process: Planning
Client Needs: Safe, Effective Care Environment
Clinical Area: Pediatric Nursing

12. (1) Direct contact with blood or body fluids from an HIV positive client is the mode of transmission. Of the situations listed, starting an IV would be the most likely way of contracting AIDS.

Nursing Process: Planning
Client Needs: Safe, Effective Care Environment
Clinical Area: Medical Nursing

13. (1) A mobile is appropriate for a 5 month old, because it provides visual stimulation. A teddy bear is not as interesting or comforting to a 5 month old as it might be to an older child. A toy that makes noise is more appropriate for ages 7 to 9 months, and it requires more motor development than a 5 month old possesses. A 5 month old does not have the fine motor development required for holding a book.

Nursing Process: Planning
Client Needs: Psychosocial Integrity
Clinical Area: Pediatric Nursing

14. (3) These hollow, muffled breath sounds can be heard over the bronchial area below the clavicle.

Nursing Process: Data Collection
Client Needs: Physiological Integrity
Clinical Area: Medical Nursing

15. (3) Auscultating lung fields provides knowledge of which lung areas are most affected. These areas should be treated first, because many clients cannot tolerate a 30-minute procedure.

Nursing Process: Implementation
Client Needs: Safe, Effective Care Environment
Clinical Area: Pediatric Nursing

16. (3) Hyperinflation of lungs with oxygen before and after suctioning prevents potential

cardiac complications due to a sudden drop in blood oxygen levels.

Nursing Process: Implementation
Client Needs: Safe, Effective Care Environment
Clinical Area: Medical Nursing

17.   (4)   The client can be turned to both sides to increase full expansion of lungs. It is best to place him in semi-Fowler's position when his vital signs are stable to ensure full lung expansion.

Nursing Process: Planning
Client Needs: Safe, Effective Care Environment
Clinical Area: Surgical Nursing

18.   (3)   A complete discharge plan provides information on nursing procedures, medications and equipment needed for care. This ensures that care is provided similarly in both settings and would contribute most to a smooth transition.

Nursing Process: Planning
Client Needs: Health Promotion and Maintenance
Clinical Area: Medical Nursing

19.   (1)   Nägele's rule is to count back 3 months from the first day of the last menstrual period and add 7 days.

Nursing Process: Planning
Client Need: Health Promotion and Maintenance
Clinical Area: Maternity Nursing

20.   (2)   A 20-degree elevation of the bed is important to maintain a patent airway and ventilation unless shock is present. Optimal positioning is every 2 hours to maintain skin integrity. Answer (1) is not specific enough, nor is answer (4). Answer (3) is incorrect because high-Fowler's position is contraindicat-

ed. The nurse would, however, rotate the client from affected to unaffected side.

Nursing Process: Planning
Client Needs: Safe, Effective Care Environment
Clinical Area: Medical Nursing

21.   (1)   A normal respiratory rate for a 1½ year old is 30 breaths/min. This rate would indicate that the child's respiratory condition is improving. The usual respiratory rate for a 14 year old is 18 breaths/min. A respiratory rate of 20 is usual for a 10 year old. A respiratory rate of 50 is abnormally high.

Nursing Process: Evaluation
Client Needs: Physiological Integrity
Clinical Area: Pediatric Nursing

22.   (3)   All drugs may be expected to cross the placental barrier and are especially damaging during the first 8 weeks, when fetal organogenesis is taking place. Drugs taken later in pregnancy may also affect the fetus, but their effects may not be known for years. Even drugs taken during labor may have a depressive effect upon the CNS of the fetus and may take several days to wear off. Nicotine from smoking may cause low birth weight infants as well as congenital defects.

Nursing Process: Implementation
Client Needs: Safe, Effective Care Environment
Clinical Area: Maternity Nursing

23.   (2)   The diet must include at least one fruit or vegetable high in vitamin C, and should include a total of four fruits and vegetables. Pregnancy requires the addition of 300 calories a day over regular caloric intake, and 1500 calories a day would be inadequate. The recommended calories for someone aged 28 are 2300 a day. New research indicates that sodium is essential, so a low sodium diet is not recommended.

Nursing Process: Implementation
Client Needs: Health Promotion and
Maintenance
Clinical Area: Maternity Nursing

24.   (4)   The state, or level, of consciousness is the most reliable index of neurological status, especially when a client has increased intracranial pressure.

   Nursing Process: Data Collection
   Client Needs: Physiological Integrity
   Clinical Area: Medical Nursing

25.   (3)   One of the most critical nursing activities for the nurse is to recognize a dangerous change in the client's condition and report it immediately.

   Nursing Process: Implementation
   Client Needs: Safe, Effective Care
   Environment
   Clinical Area: Medical Nursing

26.   (2)   Numbness of the extremities is a symptom of delayed reaction to the dye. Respiratory distress is a frequent early sign of anaphylactic shock. The release of histamine causes major vascular and bronchial symptoms resulting in anaphylaxis.

   Nursing Process: Evaluation
   Client Needs: Physiological Integrity
   Clinical Area: Surgical Nursing

27.   (3)   2000 to 3000 mL/day would be fluid maintenance postsurgery. The body will require additional fluids over the minimum due to fluid loss and the recovery process after surgery.

   Nursing Process: Planning
   Client Needs: Safe, Effective Care
   Environment
   Clinical Area: Surgical Nursing

28.   (2)   Dyspnea and tachycardia could be present due to a cardiovascular overload of fluid.

Nursing Process: Data Collection
Client Needs: Physiological Integrity
Clinical Area: Medical Nursing

29.   (1)   Edema, proteinuria and hypertension are the three cardinal signs of pre-eclampsia. Normal urine output or oliguria occurs rather than polyuria.

   Nursing Process: Data Collection
   Client Needs: Physiological Integrity
   Clinical Area: Maternity Nursing

30.   (2)   Diabetes can run in families. Obesity is a stress factor. All mothers of infants over 10 pounds should be screened for diabetes. Stillborns are common with diabetics; this is the reason so many diabetic mothers have early deliveries, often by cesarean section.

   Nursing Process: Planning
   Client Needs: Physiological Integrity
   Clinical Area: Maternity Nursing

31.   (1)   Insulin levels are increased in these infants because the mother's glucose readily crosses the placenta and stimulates the fetal pancreas to secrete increased levels of insulin. The fetal insulin does not cross the placenta.

   Nursing Process: Implementation
   Client Needs: Health Promotion and
   Maintenance
   Clinical Area: Maternity Nursing

32.   (4)   The nurse is identifying the overall feeling tone of the communication and is directly asking for feedback about her suicide potential. Most suicidal clients will give truthful information when directly asked. Answer (1) is a reflective statement and can allow her to continue talking, but it is appropriate only after her suicide potential is assessed. (2) asks for an analysis and may be distracting to the theme. (3) invalidates the client's thoughts and feelings.

Nursing Process: Implementation
Client Needs: Psychosocial Integrity
Clinical Area: Psychiatric Nursing

33. (1)   The client's plan to return home and continue therapy shows that the client has begun to realistically and responsibly deal with her problems. Talking to her boss is positive but not as comprehensive as (1). Identifying and working on weak areas usually are intermediate steps toward discharge. In asking the staff for advice, she is clearly not ready or willing to accept responsibility for herself.

    Nursing Process: Evaluation
    Client Needs: Health Promotion and Maintenance
    Clinical Area: Psychiatric Nursing

34. (4)   To promote venous return and prevent venous stasis, antigravity measures are used. Elastic hose may be worn when the client is up. Buerger-Allen exercises improve peripheral arterial circulation but are not used to promote venous return. Collateral circulation refers to the arterial system and does not aid in increasing venous return.

    Nursing Process: Planning
    Client Needs: Safe, Effective Care Environment
    Clinical Area: Medical Nursing

35. (2)   Diarrhea is a very common response to the dye tablets. A dinner of tea and toast is usually given to the client. Each dye tablet is given 5 minutes apart, usually with 1 glass of water following each tablet. The number of tablets prescribed will vary, because it is based on the weight of the client.

    Nursing Process: Implementation
    Client Needs: Safe, Effective Care Environment
    Clinical Area: Medical Nursing

36. (4)   Legg-Perthes disease affects the femoral epiphysis in which aseptic necrosis occurs. Pressure on the necrotic femur can cause permanent damage.

    Nursing Process: Planning
    Client Needs: Physiological Integrity
    Clinical Area: Pediatric Nursing

37. (2)   Fantasy is very active in this stage of development. Puppets would allow for expression of feelings. Also this activity is more active than TV or books and involves the nurse with the child, which is a positive way of establishing a relationship.

    Nursing Process: Implementation
    Client Needs: Health Promotion and Maintenance
    Clinical Area: Pediatric Nursing

38. (3)   The client's grandiose attacking statements probably reflect his feelings of fear and his anger at being afraid. Reassurance that he will be safe is important. His fear should be respected but not necessarily confronted since this might increase his anxiety. Confrontation would probably escalate his aggressiveness and add to his defensiveness. In his present state, a probing question would be threatening and inappropriate, although it might be useful later.

    Nursing Process: Implementation
    Client Needs: Safe, Effective Care Environment
    Clinical Area: Psychiatric Nursing

39. (3)   An indication of a comatose state is increased blood pressure and slowing respirations. Aphasia is also a result of increased pressure; however, due to a decreased level of consciousness which is sometimes present, this is not always an accurate indicator.

    Nursing Process: Data Collection
    Client Needs: Physiological Integrity
    Clinical Area: Medical Nursing

40. (3) All of the nursing interventions listed would be carried out for the client; however, the most important one is to prevent cerebral hypoxia (which contributes to cerebral edema) by maintaining a patent airway. The acid-base imbalance and hypoxia are often mistaken for signs of increased intracranial pressure, leading to unnecessary surgical intervention. A patent airway will establish adequate oxygenation and prevent carbon dioxide build-up.

> *Nursing Process:* Data Collection
> *Client Needs:* Safe, Effective Care Environment
> *Clinical Area:* Surgical Nursing

41. (2) Depression is more successfully treated by ECT than are the other conditions listed, and for the elderly it is safer than antidepressant drugs. A dramatic lift of the depression may be seen after only a few treatments. None of the other disorders have been found to be successfully treated with ECT.

> *Nursing Process:* Planning
> *Client Needs:* Psychosocial Integrity
> *Clinical Area:* Psychiatric Nursing

42. (1) Memory impairment is the most common side effect of ECT and has been generally shown to be temporary. None of the other symptoms are known side effects.

> *Nursing Process:* Evaluation
> *Client Needs:* Psychosocial Integrity
> *Clinical Area:* Psychiatric Nursing

43. (1) The extent of the burns is 27 percent, calculated by adding the head = 9 percent (face and neck each equal 4½ percent), arm = 9 percent, and chest = 9 percent.

> *Nursing Process:* Data Collection
> *Client Needs:* Physiological Integrity
> *Clinical Area:* Medical Nursing

44. (3) A diet high in carbohydrates is essential to allow the protein to be spared for tissue regeneration. High protein is also needed for tissue repair.

> *Nursing Process:* Planning
> *Client Needs:* Health Promotion and Maintenance
> *Clinical Area:* Medical Nursing

45. (3) This is a good opportunity for client teaching, and the first thing the nurse must do is assess the client's level of knowledge.

> *Nursing Process:* Data Collection
> *Client Needs:* Health Promotion and Maintenance
> *Clinical Area:* Medical Nursing

46. (3) A peanut butter sandwich has 12 gms of protein, more than the other foods.

> *Nursing Process:* Implementation
> *Client Needs:* Health Promotion and Maintenance
> *Clinical Area:* Maternity Nursing

47. (1) The purpose of Apgar scoring is to determine the viability of the infant. Apgar scoring is the evaluation of five vital signs: heart rate, respiratory rate, muscle tone, reflex irritability, and color. Scores of 0, 1 or 2 are given to each vital sign for a total of 10. A score of 7 to 10 is considered vigorous.

> *Nursing Process:* Planning
> *Client Needs:* Physiological Integrity
> *Clinical Area:* Maternity Nursing

48. (1) When the infant is born, he or she is wet and delivery rooms are usually cool, resulting in heat loss through conduction, convection and radiation. Placing the infant in a heated crib decreases heat loss. The Trendelenburg position is used to facilitate drainage.

Nursing Process: Planning
Client Needs: Physiological Integrity
Clinical Area: Maternity Nursing

49. (4) Infants have a weak cough and gag reflex and have difficulty removing mucus. If the bronchial secretions become dry, they are tenacious and almost impossible for the baby to expel. Secretions are also difficult to remove by suctioning. Oxygen is very drying to the mucous membranes and should always be humidified while being administered (whether to an infant or an adult).

> *Nursing Process:* Planning
> *Client Needs:* Physiological Integrity
> *Clinical Area:* Maternity Nursing

50. (2) High blood levels of oxygen cause spasms of the retinal vessels. The destruction of these vessels can cause retrolental fibroplasia resulting in blindness.

> *Nursing Process:* Evaluation
> *Client Needs:* Physiological Integrity
> *Clinical Area:* Maternity Nursing

51. (2) If there is no relief in 15 minutes, the client should notify his physician. The action of nitroglycerin is to dilate the coronary arteries to enhance blood flow to the myocardium. If the drug is not providing relief, other medical measures must be used.

> *Nursing Process:* Implementation
> *Client Needs:* Health Promotion and Maintenance
> *Clinical Area:* Medical Nursing

52. (1) Semi-Fowler's with the neck erect is the position of choice to maintain respiratory status. The objective is to decrease pressure on the suture line and prevent edema formation.

> *Nursing Process:* Implementation
> *Client Needs:* Safe, Effective Care Environment
> *Clinical Area:* Surgical Nursing

53. (1) Signs of hypoparathyroidism following a thyroidectomy are evident in an acute attack of tetany. The drug of choice is calcium gluconate to counter the low calcium level.

> *Nursing Process:* Planning
> *Client Needs:* Physiological Integrity
> *Clinical Area:* Surgical Nursing

54. (3) Due to the extreme loss of fluids from the high colon interruption, fluid and electrolyte imbalance is the most common complication. The lower colon reabsorbs a major portion of the fluid, whereas the upper colon does not have this function. A great potassium loss also occurs, because it is found in large amounts in the upper colon.

> *Nursing Process:* Evaluation
> *Client Needs:* Physiological Integrity
> *Clinical Area:* Surgical Nursing

55. (2) Corn may cause obstruction of the ileostomy and thus should be avoided. Answers (1) and (4) cause flatus and are usually avoided by clients as well.

> *Nursing Process:* Evaluation
> *Client Needs:* Health Promotion and Maintenance
> *Clinical Area:* Surgical Nursing

56. (3) Headache is often a manifestation of increased blood pressure and may indicate a worsening of his hypertension. Therefore, the safety intervention is to take the client's blood pressure so that an appropriate intervention may be made.

> *Nursing Process:* Implementation
> *Client Needs:* Safe, Effective Care Environment
> *Clinical Area:* Medical Nursing

57. (1) Positioning the client on her right side will allow pressure to be placed on the puncture site, thus promoting hemostasis.

Nursing Process: Implementation
Client Needs: Safe, Effective Care
Environment
Clinical Area: Surgical Nursing

58. (2) Any position that impedes respirations by the pressure of abdominal contents on the diaphragm should be avoided; therefore, the best position for this client is semi-Fowler's position, which increases effectiveness of breathing.

Nursing Process: Planning
Client Needs: Safe, Effective Care
Environment
Clinical Area: Medical Nursing

59. (3) In order to prevent the trauma of reinsertion, the balloons must be checked for leaks before insertion. This is done by inflating them and placing them in water to observe for bubbles. There is no mercury involved in the use of a Sengstaken-Blakemore tube.

Nursing Process: Implementation
Client Needs: Safe, Effective Care
Environment
Clinical Area: Medical Nursing

60. (2) The accumulation of phenylalanine, an amino acid breakdown of protein, is toxic to brain tissue. Therefore, any foods high in protein must be restricted. These include meat, fish, legumes, lima beans, milk products, etc.

Nursing Process: Planning
Client Needs: Health Promotion and
Maintenance
Clinical Area: Pediatric Nursing

61. (3) Blurred vision, peripheral visual loss, and an opacity are the symptoms associated with cataracts. Seeing white halos and floating spots are symptoms of a detached retina.

Nursing Process: Implementation
Client Needs: Safe, Effective Care
Environment
Clinical Area: Medical Nursing

62. (1) A prothrombin time of 30 seconds indicates the clotting time is prolonged and bleeding could occur (15 seconds is maximum normal reading). A vitamin K injection will increase the synthesis of prothrombin by the liver.

Nursing Process: Planning
Client Needs: Physiological Integrity
Clinical Area: Medical Nursing

63. (2) Carbohydrates are one of the mainstays of the cirrhotic client's diet. The liver can metabolize only very small amounts of protein, so usually only 40 to 50 grams of protein is allowed per day (normal diet is 60 to 80 grams per day). The banana is the only nonprotein choice.

Nursing Process: Evaluation
Client Needs: Health Promotion and
Maintenance
Clinical Area: Medical Nursing

64. (3) This answer orients the client to time and place in addition to assessing the underlying cause of his sleep disturbance. Answer (2) is only a short-term solution, and (4) does not focus on his problem but on other client's needs.

Nursing Process: Implementation
Client Needs: Psychosocial Integrity
Clinical Area: Psychiatric Nursing

65. (4) The advantage of an exchange diet is that it allows the client to have food such as ice cream by assessing what food groups need to be altered in order to accommodate the diet change.

Nursing Process: Implementation
Client Needs: Health Promotion and
Maintenance
Clinical Area: Pediatric Nursing

66. (1) The increase in blood pressure could cause a rupture of the aneurysm, so this finding should be reported immediately. Palpation of a pulsating mass and a bruit are normal findings. Moderate anxiety over the surgery is also normal.

    Nursing Process: Data Collection
    Client Needs: Physiological Integrity
    Clinical Area: Surgical Nursing

67. (1) It is important to recognize their grief and let them know it's normal. They need to work through their grief before they can cope with other information.

    Nursing Process: Implementation
    Client Needs: Psychosocial Integrity
    Clinical Area: Maternity Nursing

68. (3) Ophthalmia neonatorum is caused by the gonococcus organism in the birth canal. Retrolental fibroplasia is caused from a high FIO_2 delivery to premature infants. Erythroblastosis fetalis is a hemolytic disease in the newborn.

    Nursing Process: Planning
    Client Needs: Physiological Integrity
    Clinical Area: Maternity Nursing

69. (4) When a client is experiencing heart failure, the heart cannot provide for the basic needs of the body; therefore, the client is maintained on bedrest until the heart is strengthened.

    Nursing Process: Planning
    Client Needs: Health Promotion and Maintenance
    Clinical Area: Medical Nursing

70. (2) Low obstructive respiratory syndrome (bronchiolitis) has expiratory stridor with a characteristic wheeze and grunt. The respirations are rapid and shallow because of severe lung distention, but retractions are mild.

    Nursing Process: Data Collection
    Client Needs: Physiological Integrity
    Clinical Area: Pediatric Nursing

71. (2) It is important that the client be allowed to complete the ritual to reduce the anxiety. Allowing her time to do this by having her begin the ritual activity early before each meal will meet both the needs of decreasing the anxiety and good nutrition. Feeding her later would separate her from the other clients.

    Nursing Process: Implementation
    Client Needs: Psychosocial Integrity
    Clinical Area: Psychiatric Nursing

72. (4) It is important not to plan any treatment activity before or during her ritual. Immediately after completing the ritual act, the anxiety will be the lowest.

    Nursing Process: Planning
    Client Needs: Safe, Effective Care Environment
    Clinical Area: Psychiatric Nursing

73. (3) This situation involves management skills and teaching because the team leader should instruct the LVN that the NA cannot complete the necessary assessment needed for safe client care. The Foley is inserted if considerable bleeding is expected; therefore, the team leader or LVN should evaluate the drainage. If the Foley is not draining sufficiently, a complication of hemorrhage, displacement of the catheter, or perforation of the bladder during surgery might have occurred and the physician should be notified immediately. For the team leader to do the assignment herself is not appropriate because the new graduate needs guidance.

    Nursing Process: Implementation
    Client Needs: Safe, Effective Care Environment
    Clinical Area: Surgical Nursing

74. (2) As acetone is liberated through the breakdown of fat, it is volatile and is blown off by the lungs, creating the characteristic fruity odor of the breath. Polyuria (not oliguria), polydipsia, and polyphagia are early symptoms.

> *Nursing Process:* Data Collection
> *Client Needs:* Physiological Integrity
> *Clinical Area:* Medical Nursing

75. (2) The position of choice is the left side because of the anatomical position of the colon. Sims' position will facilitate instillation.

> *Nursing Process:* Implementation
> *Client Needs:* Safe, Effective Care Environment
> *Clinical Area:* Medical Nursing

76. (3) Infants begin to sit with support or leaning forward on both hands at 6 months. They sit with minimal or no support between 7 and 8 months. If this milestone does not occur, the infant should be assessed for retardation.

> *Nursing Process:* Data Collection
> *Client Needs:* Health Promotion and Maintenance
> *Clinical Area:* Pediatric Nursing

77. (4) Hemophilia is a sex-linked recessive disorder. The asymptomatic mother transmits the disorder to the son on the X chromosome.

> *Nursing Process:* Planning
> *Client Needs:* Physiological Integrity
> *Clinical Area:* Pediatric Nursing

78. (2) Regurgitation or spitting up can be caused by feeding too much formula at one time or the need for more burping, and usually diminishes by 5 or 6 months. Reducing the amount of each feeding may be sufficient to stop the problem. A nipple with a large opening, not a small one, can cause regurgitation.

> *Nursing Process:* Implementation
> *Client Needs:* Safe, Effective Care Environment
> *Clinical Area:* Pediatric Nursing

79. (1) The major goal of treatment is prevention of permanent cardiac damage. Penicillin treats the streptococcal infection. Aspirin relieves joint pain and decreases the temperature.

> *Nursing Process:* Planning
> *Client Needs:* Physiological Integrity
> *Clinical Area:* Pediatric Nursing

80. (2) The aim of the public health department is to immunize 80 percent of the population. This number will protect the remaining 20 percent.

> *Nursing Process:* Planning
> *Client Needs:* Health Promotion and Maintenance
> *Clinical Area:* Pediatric Nursing

81. (3) It is the nurse's responsibility to inform the charge nurse or supervisor about the observation. Stealing drugs is obviously illegal, but the administration should handle reporting it to the authorities.

> *Nursing Process:* Implementation
> *Client Needs:* Safe, Effective Care Environment
> *Clinical Area:* Psychiatric Nursing

82. (1) Cogentin or Artane are the antiparkinson drugs usually prescribed for reducing extrapyramidal effects caused by phenothiazines. Benadryl is also commonly used and has fewer side effects. The other answers are incorrect—Niamid and Ritalin are antidepressant drugs and Valium is classified as an antianxiety drug.

> *Nursing Process:* Planning
> *Client Needs:* Physiological Integrity
> *Clinical Area:* Psychiatric Nursing

83.   (3)   Contact either the poison control center or the emergency department first and follow their instructions. In this case they will probably advise giving the child water to dilute the ferrous sulfate tablets and syrup of ipecac to induce vomiting. Because some poisons will be damaging if vomited, the center would not always advise the mother to give syrup of ipecac. Then the nurse would instruct the mother to bring the child to the hospital.

Nursing Process: Implementation
Client Needs: Safe, Effective Care Environment
Clinical Area: Pediatric Nursing

84.   (3)   The client is experiencing side effects to phenothiazines, but these are not life-threatening and can be brought to the attention of the head nurse and physician within an appropriate amount of time. (4) is incorrect. Thorazine is effective at certain blood levels, and holding the drug would lower the blood level. If possible, it is preferable to check with the physician before holding a drug.

Nursing Process: Implementation
Client Needs: Safe, Effective Care Environment
Clinical Area: Psychiatric Nursing

85.   (3)   For a left hemisphere lesion, the best method of communication is to pantomime what you are communicating while speaking in a normal tone of voice. Pantomime will confuse a person who has suffered a right hemisphere lesion. Before communicating, however, the nurse will assess the client's ability to understand speech. It is also important to give feedback as you communicate.

Nursing Process: Planning
Client Needs: Psychosocial Integrity
Clinical Area: Medical Nursing

86.   (3)   The clinical manifestations are typical of gallbladder disease and thus the nurse would continue to follow admission orders. This client does not require additional fluid at this time.

Nursing Process: Implementation
Client Needs: Safe, Effective Care Environment
Clinical Area: Medical Nursing

87.   (4)   Nervous control for the diaphragm (phrenic nerve) exists at the level of C_3 or C_4 of the spinal cord.

Nursing Process: Planning
Client Needs: Physiological Integrity
Clinical Area: Surgical Nursing

88.   (4)   GI bleeding is a very common complication associated with portal hypertension. Obstruction of portal circulation leads to increased collateral circulation which can result in bleeding tendencies.

Nursing Process: Data Collection
Client Needs: Physiological Integrity
Clinical Area: Medical Nursing

89.   (3)   In organic brain disorder, barbiturates commonly cause delirium, confusion, and paradoxical excitement, thus they should not be ordered for clients with organic brain disorder.

Nursing Process: Planning
Client Needs: Physiological Integrity
Clinical Area: Psychiatric Nursing

90.   (3)   Intermediate insulin peaks from 8 to 12 hours after injection. 3:30 PM is the most appropriate time to assess for signs of insulin reaction.

Nursing Process: Evaluation
Client Needs: Physiological Integrity
Clinical Area: Medical Nursing

IV

SELF-ASSESSMENT AND EVALUATION GRIDS

COMPREHENSIVE TESTS 1 & 2

Self-Assessment and Evaluation Grids

Introduction

The purpose of this section—self-assessment and evaluation—is to assist you to direct your own review based on your individual needs. After you complete the comprehensive tests, you can utilize the following grids to determine your specific areas of competence as well as your areas of vulnerability. The self-study suggestions will assist you to correct your deficient areas. This process should increase your confidence regarding the NCLEX CAT.

The self-assessment grids explained on the following pages are designed to provide you with helpful feedback. If you have a short period of time to prepare for your licensure exam, it is important that you promptly identify topics requiring further review and study. These assessment and evaluation grids will enable you to assess weak areas and evaluate your strengths so that you will be able to focus your additional review systematically and efficiently.

Use the grids as a tool to diagnose probable areas of weakness by assessing where you answered most questions incorrectly. If in reviewing those areas you feel confident with your knowledge base, reread the questions you answered incorrectly, then read the rationale to determine why you chose the wrong answer. Perhaps you misunderstood the question or simply forgot something you once knew, such as the pharmacological action of a drug. *It is important to pinpoint your specific weaknesses so that you can prioritize your learning objectives and design a study program.*

After completing the assessment and evaluation grids for Comprehensive Tests 1 and 2 and your self-study program, review the nursing content areas where you feel the weakest. Complete the individual clinical questions and again check for areas of weakness. Next, complete the final two comprehensive tests and assessment grids. You should be scoring more than 60% correct. Use the computer disk accompanying this book to further test your mastery of nursing content. This disk is designed to increase your confidence concerning computer testing. As you gain more experience with answering questions presented on screen and practice under simulated test conditions, your comfort level and, hence, confidence should increase. After taking the test on the disk, you can obtain a computer-generated Performance Summary. This feedback will include your results in terms of Nursing Process, Client Needs and Clinical Area. These results will indicate areas of relative weakness where you can focus further study and review.

General Directions for Using Self-Assessment Grids

The Comprehensive Tests cover all areas of practical nursing. In order for you to complete a self-assessment and identify your deficient areas of nursing knowledge, it is necessary to categorize the questions. Thus, the five areas of clinical practice are included in each grid: medical nursing, surgical nursing, pediatric nursing, maternity nursing, and psychiatric nursing. As you will note after completing all four Comprehensive Tests, the five clinical areas are quite evenly dispersed throughout.

Because the NCLEX Test Plan is essentially oriented around the Nursing Process and Client Needs, the self-assessment grids follow a similar focus. Grid I enables you to list the questions you missed in terms of Nursing Process and Clinical Area. To complete Grid II, you will record your missed questions in terms of Client Needs and Clinical Area.

1. Complete Comprehensive Tests 1 and 2.

2. Write the number of the questions answered incorrectly on Grids I and II.

3. After you have recorded your incorrect answers, total them and enter the number in the Total Answers Wrong column on each grid. Add the total for Grids I and II.

4. Now complete your self-assessment by following the directions in the section **Prioritizing Topics for Further Review**.

5. After you have studied material relating to your weak areas and completed the individual clinical area questions, complete Comprehensive Tests 3 and 4.

6. Repeat steps #2 to 4 on grids in section VII.

Grid I   Nursing Process/Clinical Area

The focus of this grid is to assess your ability to answer questions reflecting the nursing process. The questions are categorized according to the following steps.

Data Collection: This phase in the nursing process requires skilled observation, reasoning, and a theoretical knowledge base to differentiate data, verify data, and document findings. This phase also includes identification of client needs, formulation of client goals with priorities for goal achievement, and the nursing diagnoses.

Planning: This phase refers to the identification of nursing actions which are strategies to achieve the established goals. This phase also includes nursing measures for the delivery of care. Clients and other health team members may be involved in the planning phase.

Implementation: This phase refers to the priority nursing action or interventions performed to accomplish a specified goal. Nursing actions center on implementing the plan of care (to achieve a goal).

Evaluation: Dependent on the previous steps of the nursing process, this phase determines the extent to which goals are accomplished. This step completes the Nursing Process and determines if the nursing action was appropriate and goals were achieved. If the goals were not achieved, a re-examination of the steps of nursing process is completed to identify at which phase there is a need for change.

Grid II   Client Needs/Clinical Area

After filling out Grid II, you will be able to identify your areas of relative weakness in terms of Client Needs. The National Council of State Boards of Nursing has defined the entry level nurse's job tasks as providing for four essential Client Needs: (1) Safe, effective care environment, (2) Physiological integrity, (3) Psychosocial integrity, and (4) Health promotion and maintenance. Additional description of Client Needs and their subcategories is contained in Part I, Preparing for the NCLEX-PN.

Prioritizing Topics for Further Review

1. After completing the grids, you will have a general indication of your deficient areas.

2. Identify weak areas by determining in which sections you have the most incorrect answers in descending order. List your weakest areas of knowledge first.

3. This is an overview of potentially vulnerable areas in which you may require further review.

4. Note any patterns you see developing. For example, do you have many incorrect answers in the implementation phase of the nursing process, the clinical discipline of medicine, the client needs of safe, effective care environment? If so, this pattern would direct you to begin your review in these areas: the client need for safe, effective care within the discipline of medicine, with a focus on implementation.

5. Now, prioritize and focus on these topics for further study and review.

6. The best resource to assist you to review in an efficient manner is an NCLEX review book in which the material is presented in a concise and comprehensive format. A recommended review book is ***Content Review for the NCLEX-PN,*** also by Sandra Smith, RN, MS. This book is organized by clinical area and nursing process.

7. After you have completed additional study and review, answer the questions organized by subject area.

    a. After further review, do you now feel more comfortable with the material?

    b. Did you score relatively high (between 60 and 70 percent correct) on the subject area exams?

    c. If your score was lower than 60 percent on any of the subject area tests, then it would be useful to do more review in that area.

8. Next, answer all the questions in Comprehensive Tests 3 and 4.

9. Fill out the assessment and evaluation grids that follow Test 4. Record and total the incorrect answers. You should be achieving higher scores on these tests.

10. Fill out the chart on the next page and check your results on Tests 3 and 4 against Tests 1 and 2. Is there a consistent pattern in your areas of relative weakness?

11. Finally, you should complete the Comprehensive Test on the disk enclosed with this book. These questions were not included in the book, so you will be able to take a new test and obtain a detailed Performance Summary. Compare your results on the computer disk to your earlier grids. If your study and review sessions have been effective, your Performance Summary percentages should show your progress. If not, you may need further review. Find more practice questions in other NCLEX review books. Continue to identify your weak areas and review this material again until you feel confident.

Comprehensive Tests 1 & 2

Grid I—Nursing Process   Grid I—Clinical Area   Grid II—Client Needs

_____   _____   _____

_____   _____   _____

_____   _____   _____

_____   _____   _____

Comprehensive Tests 3 & 4

Grid I—Nursing Process   Grid I—Clinical Area   Grid II—Client Needs

_____   _____   _____

_____   _____   _____

_____   _____   _____

_____   _____   _____

Grid I Comprehensive Texts 1 & 2	Clinical Area					
	Medical Nursing	Surgical Nursing	Maternity Nursing	Pediatric Nursing	Psychiatric Nursing	Total Answers Wrong
Data Collection						
Planning						
Implementation						
Evaluation						
Total Answers Wrong						

Nursing Process

Grid II Comprehensive Texts 1 & 2		Clinical Area					
		Medical Nursing	**Surgical Nursing**	**Maternity Nursing**	**Pediatric Nursing**	**Psychiatric Nursing**	**Total Answers Wrong**
Client Needs	**Safe, Effective Care Environment**						
	Physiological Integrity						
	Psychosocial Integrity						
	Health Promotion and Maintenance						
	Total Answers Wrong						

V

CLINCIAL AREA Q&A

MEDICAL-SURGICAL NURSING

MEDICAL QUESTIONS

1. The nurse has an order to remove a client's nasogastric tube. The correct nursing action related to this procedure would be to

   1 Put on sterile gloves after untaping the tube from the client's face.
   2 Instill 30 mL of normal saline before removing the tube.
   3 Pull the tube out slowly and gently.
   4 Pull the tube out quickly while keeping it pinched.

2. What size needle should be used to administer an intramuscular dose of meperidine (Demerol) to an adult client?

   1 18 gauge.
   2 20 gauge.
   3 22 gauge.
   4 25 gauge.

3. The LVN's primary responsibility in monitoring IV therapy is to

   1 Frequently check and regulate the flow of solution according to the amount ordered.
   2 Monitor frequently so that the IV remains open and add a new bottle of solution if necessary.
   3 Record accurate IV intake for the shift.
   4 Change the IV site every 24 hours to prevent collapse of the vein.

4. The nurse knows there is a need for further teaching when the client taking Coumadin says

   1 "I cannot eat foods high in vitamin K, such as leafy vegetables."
   2 "I can take aspirin for my 'aches and pains'."

   3 "I need to have a prothrombin time before I return to the doctor."
   4 "I need to report any bleeding to the doctor."

5. The nurse is teaching an insulin-dependent diabetic client to self-test her blood glucose. The nurse tells her that if she obtains a result that is over 250 mg/dL, she should

   1 Test her urine for ketones.
   2 Reduce the amount of food that she eats.
   3 Increase her dose of regular insulin by 5 units.
   4 Do nothing unless the results remain elevated for 2 days.

6. A person who is infected with HIV will be diagnosed with AIDS when the CD4 lymphocyte count falls below

   1 75.
   2 200.
   3 350.
   4 500.

7. The nurse will know that the client on a sodium restricted diet needs more teaching after hearing which of the following statements?

   1 "I must check food labels for preservatives."
   2 "I must check labels on any over-the-counter drugs I use."
   3 "I can drink all the milk I want."
   4 I can eat all the fresh fruits and vegetables I want."

8. A client is experiencing tachycardia. The nurse's understanding of the physiological basis for this symptom is explained by which of the following statements?

1 The demand for oxygen is decreased because of pleural involvement.

2 The inflammatory process causes the body to demand more oxygen to meet its needs.

3 The heart has to pump faster to meet the demand for oxygen when there is lowered arterial oxygen tension.

4 Respirations are labored.

9. Which nursing diagnosis should receive highest priority in a client who is receiving the chemotherapeutic agent cisplatin (Platinol)?

1 Risk of infection.

2 Activity intolerance.

3 Altered oral mucous membranes.

4 Altered nutrition: less than body requirements.

10. A client in hepatic coma has orders for phenobarbital. The nurse knows that this drug is preferred to a depressant drug because it is

1 Excreted by the kidney.

2 Not as strong as a depressant drug.

3 Relaxing for an agitated client.

4 Safe when the blood ammonia level is up.

11. A female client with a tentative diagnosis of urinary tract infection has been admitted to the unit. The nurse knows that the most important factor influencing ascending infection is

1 Not enough fluid intake.

2 Obstruction of free urine flow.

3 A change in pH.

4 Presence of micro-organisms.

12. When administering a tepid bath to reduce a client's temperature, the client begins to shiver. The intervention would be to

1 Continue with the bath, as this helps dissipate the heat.

2 Stop the bath briefly and place a warm blanket on the client to stop shivering.

3 Stop the bath, as the body is attempting to produce heat.

4 Warm the solution, continue the bath, and change the location of cloth placement.

13. A client is about to be discharged on the drug bishydroxycoumarin (Dicumarol). Of the principles below, which one is the most important to teach the client before discharge?

1 He should be sure to take the medication before meals.

2 He should shave with an electric razor.

3 If he misses a dose, he should double the dose at the next scheduled time.

4 It is the responsibility of the RN to do the teaching for this medication.

14. The client with myasthenia gravis is being treated with an anticholinergic drug, neostigmine (Prostigmin). In administering this drug, the most important nursing measure is to

1 Give the medication exactly on time.

2 Give the medication with plenty of water.

3 Monitor the client's intake and output.

4 Monitor the client's vital signs before and after the medication.

15. The LVN is teaching a nursing assistant to remove a pair of used gloves. The LVN would demonstrate to remove the first glove by

1 Grasping the outer surface of the cuff with the other hand and pulling the glove off while turning it inside out.

2 Placing several fingers of the other hand inside the wrist of the first glove and pulling it off while turning it inside out.

3 Grasping the ends of several fingers with the other hand and pulling the glove straight off.

4 Rolling the glove down to the palm using the other hand, then placing a finger inside the rolled glove and pulling it off.

16. A cyanotic client with an unknown diagnosis is admitted to the emergency room. In relation to oxygen, the first nursing action would be to

    1 Wait until the client's lab work is done.
    2 Not administer oxygen unless ordered by the physician.
    3 Administer oxygen at 2 liters flow per minute.
    4 Administer oxygen at 10 liters flow per minute and check the client's nail beds.

17. A client is started on ASA therapy. She tells the nurse that she is having a great deal of gastrointestinal distress. The therapeutic response would be to

    1 Inform the charge nurse so the physician can change to another drug.
    2 Explain that this happens frequently and there is nothing to be concerned about.
    3 Ask the client when she takes the drug during the day.
    4 Tell the client to take an antacid with the drug.

18. A client with a diagnosis of gout will be taking colchicine and allopurinol bid to prevent recurrence. The most common early sign of colchicine toxicity that the nurse will observe for is

    1 Blurred vision.
    2 Anorexia.
    3 Diarrhea.
    4 Fever.

19. An employee at the local factory comes to the nurse's office with a large furuncle (boil) on his left upper arm. He has come to the office with this same complaint over the past 6 months. In addition to specific care for the boil itself, the nursing intervention should include

    1 Advising the client to bathe more regularly.
    2 Doing nothing else, as furuncles are not related to any other disease process.

3 Calling in all employees and checking them for furuncles.
    4 Encouraging the client to see his family physician as recurrent boils may be a sign of underlying disease.

20. The nurse is inserting a Foley catheter into a male client. How far should the catheter be inserted before inflating the balloon?

    1 3 to 4 inches.
    2 5 to 6 inches.
    3 7 to 9 inches.
    4 10 to 12 inches.

21. The importance of providing instructions to women on self-examination of the breast is best reflected in which of the following statements?

    1 The majority of breast abnormalities are first discovered by women.
    2 Once a lesion has been discovered, the informed client may monitor the progress of the abnormality herself.
    3 Breast cancer occurs much more often in women than men and is a major cause of death in women.
    4 The high mortality rate of breast cancer can be most effectively reduced by early detection and adequate surgical treatment.

22. Which of the following complications of acute bacterial endocarditis would the nurse constantly observe for in an acutely ill client?

    1 Presence of a heart murmur.
    2 Emboli.
    3 Fever.
    4 Congestive heart failure.

23. A 53-year-old female client has returned to the unit following a laparoscopic cholecystectomy. She complains of right shoulder pain. The nurse would explain to the client that this pain is

1 Common following this type of operation.
2 Expected after general anesthesia.
3 Unusual and will be reported to the surgeon.
4 Indicative of a need to use the incentive spirometer.

24. The nurse would chart that a client is experiencing Cheyne-Stokes respiration when he has

1 Periods of hyperpnea alternating with periods of apnea.
2 Periods of tachypnea alternating with periods of apnea.
3 An increase in both rate and depth of respirations.
4 Deep, regular, sighing respirations.

25. Basilar crackles are present in a client's lungs on auscultation. The nurse knows that these are discrete, noncontinuous sounds that are

1 Caused by the sudden opening of alveoli.
2 Usually more prominent during expiration.
3 Produced by air flow across passages narrowed by secretions.
4 Found primarily in the pleura.

26. In developing a nursing care plan for a client with Buerger's disease, it is important to include

1 Buerger-Allen exercises.
2 Exercises to increase collateral circulation.
3 Thigh high TEDs at all times.
4 Side effects of drug therapy.

27. The nurse is collecting data on a client with joint pain. The nurse knows that a client who is in the early stages of rheumatoid arthritis is most likely to complain of pain, swelling and limitation of motion in the

1 Hips.
2 Knees.
3 Hands.
4 Spine.

28. The nurse would expect to find an improvement in which of the blood values as a result of dialysis treatment?

1 High serum creatinine levels.
2 Low hemoglobin.
3 Hypocalcemia.
4 Hypokalemia.

29. A 50-year-old client has a tracheostomy and requires tracheal suctioning. The first intervention in completing this procedure would be to

1 Change the tracheostomy dressing.
2 Provide humidity with a trach mask.
3 Apply oral or nasal suction.
4 Deflate the tracheal cuff.

30. The exercise that would be most beneficial for a client with COPD is

1 Controlled coughing.
2 Whistling while exhaling.
3 Deep breathing.
4 Incentive spirometry.

31. The nurse is teaching a Type I diabetic client about her diet, which is based on the exchange system. The nurse will know the client has learned correctly when she says that she can have as much as she wants of

1 Lettuce.
2 Tomato.
3 Grapefruit juice.
4 Skim milk.

32. The nurse notices that a client on a medical unit is alone in his room and crying. The most therapeutic nursing approach would be to say

1 "Don't cry, you'll just feel worse."
2 "Cheer up now—crying can make you feel more sad."

3 "Spending so much time alone makes one feel lonely—let's go out on the unit."

4 "I'll get a tissue and then come back and sit with you."

33. A client has sustained multiple injuries and fractures in a motor vehicle accident (MVA). During which period would the nurse be most vigilant in observing for the development of a fat embolism?

1 During the first 24 to 48 hours after the MVA.

2 72 to 96 hours after the MVA.

3 During the first week after the MVA.

4 During the second week after the MVA.

34. A client with an admitting diagnosis of head injury has a Glasgow Coma Score of 3 - 5 - 4. The nurse's understanding of this test is that the client

1 Can follow simple commands.

2 Will make no attempt to vocalize.

3 Is unconscious.

4 Is able to open his eyes when spoken to.

35. The nursing diagnosis that would have the highest priority in the care of a client who has become comatose following a cerebral hemorrhage is

1 Impaired physical mobility.

2 Altered nutrition: less than body requirements.

3 Ineffective airway clearance.

4 Constipation.

36. Part of a plan of care for a client with increased intracranial pressure is to maintain an adequate airway and to promote gas exchange. To accomplish these goals, an effective nursing action is to

1 Encourage the client to cough vigorously.

2 Avoid hypercapnia in the client.

3 Suction the client nasotracheally at frequent intervals.

4 Pack gauze in the nares when there is drainage from the nose.

37. The client has orders for Nitropaste Ointment, 1 inch every 6 hours. He complains of a headache after each application. The nursing intervention is to

1 Check the blood pressure for hypertension.

2 Decrease the dose to ¾ inch.

3 Give an analgesic such as acetaminophen (Tylenol) as ordered PRN.

4 Only apply the paste every 8 hours.

38. Based on nursing knowledge, the nurse is aware that an epidural hematoma is characterized by

1 A long period of unconsciousness followed by complete lucidity.

2 A short period of unconsciousness followed by a lucid period, followed by rapid deterioration.

3 Slowly developing signs of increasing intracranial pressure.

4 No complaints of headaches.

39. The nurse would determine that a thrombus is present by testing for

1 Doll's sign.

2 Kernig's sign.

3 Hegar's sign.

4 Homan's sign.

40. A client is admitted following an automobile accident in which he sustained a contusion. The nurse knows that the significance of a contusion is that

1 It is reversible.

2 Amnesia will occur.

3 Loss of consciousness may be transient.

4 Laceration of the brain may occur.

41. The major rationale for the use of acetylsalicylic acid (aspirin) in the treatment of rheumatoid arthritis is to

1 Reduce fever.
2 Reduce inflammation of the joints.
3 Assist the client in range-of-motion activities without pain.
4 Prevent extension of the disease process.

42. A client with chronic lymphocytic leukemia is started on chemotherapy. Monitoring the administration of these drugs, the nurse would

1 Offer a liquid diet before the treatments.
2 Offer fluids and foods high in bulk and fiber several hours before the treatment.
3 Encourage the client to eat a high starch meal just before the treatment.
4 Encourage large, rather than small, frequent meals.

43. Lactulose is ordered for a 68-year-old client hospitalized with hepatic failure. The nurse knows that the primary action of this drug is to

1 Prevent constipation.
2 Decrease the blood ammonia level.
3 Increase intestinal peristalsis.
4 Prevent portal hypertension.

44. The major goal of therapy when Dexa-metha-sone (Decadron) is ordered for a client is to

1 Replace adrenocorticoids in clients following adrenalectomy.
2 Decrease inflammation in cerebral edema.
3 Reverse signs and symptoms of septic shock.
4 Delay complications of hepatic coma in cirrhosis clients.

45. In developing a nursing care plan for a client with multiple sclerosis, the nurse would *not* include

1 Preventative measures for falls.
2 Interventions to promote bowel elimination.

3 Instructions on doing only moderate activities.
4 Techniques to promote safe swallowing.

46. Which one of the following conditions could lead to an inaccurate pulse oximetry reading if the sensor is attached to the client's ear?

1 Artificial nails.
2 Vasodilation.
3 Hypothermia.
4 Movement of the head.

47. Client education is an important component of the total nursing care plan. The primary purpose of client education is to

1 Collect client data.
2 Determine readiness to learn.
3 Assess degree of compliance.
4 Increase client's knowledge that will affect health status.

48. Thrombolytic therapy would be appropriate for which of the following conditions?

1 Continual blood pressure above 200/120.
2 History of diabetic retinopathy.
3 History of significant kidney disease.
4 Myocardial infarction.

49. While on a camping trip, a friend sustains a snake bite from a poisonous snake. The most effective initial intervention would be to

1 Place a restrictive band above the snake bite.
2 Elevate the bite area above the level of the heart.
3 Position the client in a supine position.
4 Immobilize the limb.

50. Which one of the following rules for charting narrative notes does not fit into acceptable charting procedures?

1 Each entry should be signed with the nurse's name and professional status.

2 Objective facts are more relevant than nursing interpretation.

3 Behaviors rather than feelings should be charted.

4 Use of the word "client" or "patient" is important to designate particular entries.

51. There is a physician's order to irrigate a client's bladder. Which one of the following nursing measures will ensure patency?

1 Use a solution of sterile water for the irrigation.

2 Apply a small amount of pressure to push the mucus out of the catheter tip if the tube is not patent.

3 Carefully insert about 100 mL of aqueous Zephiran into the bladder, allow it to remain for 1 hour, and then siphon it out.

4 Irrigate with 20 mLs of normal saline to establish patency.

52. When assessing an ECG, the nurse knows that the P-R interval represents the time it takes for the

1 Impulse to begin atrial contraction.

2 Impulse to traverse the atria to the AV node.

3 SA node to discharge the impulse to begin atrial depolarization.

4 Impulse to travel to the ventricles.

53. When a client has suffered severe burns all over his body, the most effective method of monitoring the cardiovascular system is

1 Cuff blood pressure.

2 Arterial pressure.

3 Central venous pressure.

4 Pulmonary artery pressure.

54. A female client has orders for an oral cholecystogram. Prior to the test, the nursing intervention would be to

1 Provide a high fat diet for dinner, then NPO.

2 Explain that diarrhea may result from the dye tablets.

3 Administer the dye tablets following a regular diet for dinner.

4 Administer enemas until clear.

55. The practical nurse knows there is a need for further teaching when the hemodialysis client with an arteriovenous fistula in the left arm says

1 "I can carry heavy packages in my right arm.

2 "You cannot take my blood pressure in my left arm."

3 "I can wear several bracelets to cover the scar on my left arm."

4 "You can start the IV in my right arm."

56. Knowing that a client has the diagnosis of congestive heart failure (CHF), what symptoms would the nurse check out in data collection?

1 Crackles, bradycardia, arrhythmias.

2 Cyanosis, crackles, gallop rhythm.

3 Anxiety, bronchospasm, pedal edema.

4 Diaphoresis, orthopnea, sensorium changes.

57. Moving a client from the bed to a chair, the first intervention is to

1 Dangle the client at his bedside.

2 Put nonslip shoes or slippers on client's feet.

3 Rock the client and pivot.

4 Position client so that he is comfortable.

58. When a client has peptic ulcer disease, the nurse would expect a priority intervention to be

1 Assisting in inserting a Miller-Abbott tube.

2 Assisting in inserting an arterial pressure line.

3 Inserting a nasogastric tube.

4 Inserting an IV.

59. Following surgery, a client has an IV of D$_5$W to run 50 mL/hour. When the nurse checks his condition for the evening shift, she realizes the IV is 1 hour behind. The first action would be to

1　Increase the flow rate to make up for the loss within the next 2 to 3 hours.
2　Continue IV flow at the same rate.
3　Increase the flow so that the loss is made up over the remaining hours in the day.
4　Notify the physician for new orders to decrease the 24-hour total fluid intake.

60. The nurse is assigned to draw blood from a suspected AIDS client. Universal precautions dictate that she should use

1　Gown, clean gloves, and mask.
2　Gown, sterile gloves.
3　Handwashing, gown, clean gloves.
4　Handwashing, sterile gloves.

61. When the nurse is completing an assessment of a burned client, second-degree burns would appear as

1　Full thickness with extension to underlying muscle and bone.
2　Partial thickness with erythema and often edema, but no vesicles.
3　Partial thickness with involvement of epidermis and dermis, showing edema and vesicles.
4　Full thickness with dry, waxy, or leathery appearance without vesicles.

62. A client with pulmonary edema is admitted to the unit. Which of the following physician's orders should the nurse question?

1　Administer furosemide (Lasix) 20 mg IV immediately.
2　Administer oxygen at 3 liters per minute via nasal prongs.
3　Keep the head of the client's bed in low-Fowler's position.
4　Weigh the client every day.

63. In preparation for discharge of a client with arterial insufficiency and Raynaud's disease, client teaching instructions should include

1　Walking several times each day as part of an exercise routine.
2　Keeping the heat up so that the environment is warm.
3　Wearing TED hose during the day.
4　Using hydrotherapy for increasing oxygenation.

64. Assessing the urine of a client with suspected cholecystitis, the nurse expects that the color will most likely be

1　Pale yellow.
2　Greenish-brown.
3　Red.
4　Yellow-orange.

65. The treatment prescribed for the burned area of skin before skin grafting can take place will include

1　Silver nitrate soaks for 24 hours.
2　Burn irrigations with Sulfamylon.
3　Warm soaks with sterile water.
4　Germicidal soap scrubs to the affected area.

66. When a client asks the nurse why the physician says he "thinks" the client has tuberculosis, the nurse explains to him that diagnosis of tuberculosis can take several weeks to confirm. Which of the following statements supports this answer?

1　A positive reaction to a tuberculosis skin test indicates that the client has active tuberculosis, even if one negative sputum is obtained.
2　A positive sputum culture takes at least 3 weeks, due to the slow reproduction of the bacillus.
3　Because small lesions are hard to detect on chest x-rays, x-rays usually need to be

repeated during several consecutive weeks.

4 A client with a positive smear will have to have a positive culture to confirm the diagnosis.

67. The nurse is counseling a client with the diagnosis of glaucoma. She explains that if left untreated, this condition leads to

1 Blindness.
2 Myopia.
3 Retrolental fibroplasia.
4 Uveitis.

68. A client is admitted with a diagnosis of esophageal varices. When collecting data, the nurse will expect to find which of the following conditions that contributed to the diagnosis?

1 Decreased prothrombin formation.
2 Decreased albumin formation by the liver.
3 Portal hypertension.
4 Increased central venous pressure.

69. A nursing assessment for initial signs of hypoglycemia will include

1 Pallor, blurred vision, weakness, behavioral changes.
2 Frequent urination, flushed face, pleural friction rub.
3 Abdominal pain, diminished deep tendon reflexes, double vision.
4 Weakness, lassitude, irregular pulse, dilated pupils.

70. One of the major goals of therapy for a client with peptic ulcer disease is to

1 Talk about the recent stressful situations which may have contributed to the ulcer formation.
2 Understand the pathogenesis of the ulcer.
3 Accept that stress will negatively affect the condition.
4 Discover what foods caused pain.

71. The physician has ordered a 24-hour urine specimen. After explaining the procedure to the client, the nurse collects the first specimen. This specimen is then

1 Discarded, then the collection begins.
2 Saved as part of the 24-hour collection.
3 Tested, then discarded.
4 Placed in a separate container and later added to the collection.

72. When a head injury client has fluid draining from the left ear, the nurse will immediately position the client with the head of his bed

1 Elevated and his head turned to the left.
2 Flat and his head turned to the right.
3 Flat and his head turned to the left.
4 Elevated and his head turned to the right.

73. As the nurse is completing evening care for a client, he observes that the client is upset, quiet and withdrawn. The nurse knows that the client is scheduled for diagnostic tests the following day. An important question to ask the client is

1 "Would you like to go to the dayroom to watch TV?"
2 "Are you prepared for the test tomorrow?"
3 "Have you talked with anyone about the test tomorrow?"
4 "Have you asked your physician to give you a sleeping pill tonight?"

74. Assessing a client's shunt for patency by using a stethoscope and the nurse's hand, the nurse would expect to feel and hear

1 A loud bruit and feel the area cool to touch.
2 The sound of rushing blood and feel the area warm to touch.
3 No sound, but feel the area warm to touch.
4 A regular heartbeat and feel the area cool to touch.

75. A male client complaining of persistent lower back pain for several months has been admitted for a work-up prior to a laminectomy. After a myelogram, which uses a water soluble dye, the nurse will position him in a

1 Side-lying position.
2 Supine position with the head of the bed elevated.
3 Dorsal recumbent position with the head flat.
4 Prone position.

76. The most appropriate nursing intervention for a client requiring a finger probe pulse oximeter is to

1 Apply the sensor probe over a finger and cover lightly with gauze to prevent skin breakdown.
2 Set alarms on the oximeter to at least 100 percent.
3 Identify if the client has had a recent diagnostic test using intravenous dye.
4 Remove the sensor between oxygen saturation readings.

77. A female client is admitted with a diagnosis of seizure disorder. A priority in protecting the client against injury during a seizure is to

1 Restrain her arms so that she won't hit herself.
2 Use a padded tongue blade so that she won't injure her tongue.
3 Keep her on her back so that she can breathe.
4 Position her on her side to facilitate drainage.

78. When a client is in liver failure, which of the following behavioral changes is the most important assessment to report?

1 Shortness of breath.
2 Lethargy.
3 Fatigue.
4 Nausea.

79. A 55-year-old client with severe epigastric pain due to acute pancreatitis has been admitted to the hospital. The client's activity at this time should be

1 Ambulation as desired.
2 Bedrest in supine position.
3 Up ad lib and right side-lying position in bed.
4 Bedrest in Fowler's position.

80. A 25-year old female client with a lower urinary tract infection is admitted to the hospital. Her history indicates she has suffered from repeated infections. The initial data collection will most likely reveal

1 Frequency and dysuria.
2 Fever and chills.
3 Malodorous, cloudy urine.
4 Leukocytosis and back pain.

81. The most common cause of bladder infection in the client with a retention catheter is contamination

1 Due to insertion technique.
2 At the time of catheter removal.
3 Of the urethral/catheter interface.
4 Of the internal lumen of the catheter.

82. The nurse will know a client with lupus erythematosus understands principles of self-care when she can discuss

1 Drying agents.
2 Moisturizing agents.
3 Antifungal creams.
4 Solar protection.

83. A client in acute renal failure receives an IV infusion of 10% dextrose in water with 20 units of regular insulin. The nurse understands that the rationale for this therapy is to

1 Correct the hyperglycemia that occurs with acute renal failure.

2 Facilitate the intracellular movement of potassium.

3 Provide calories to prevent tissue catabolism and azotemia.

4 Force potassium into the cells to prevent arrhythmias.

84. A client in the early stages of progressive renal failure is admitted to the hospital. The initial assessment will probably reveal

1 Oliguria, nausea, elevated urine specific gravity.

2 Anuria, weight gain, hypertension.

3 Polyuria, low urine specific gravity, polydipsia.

4 Hematuria, proteinuria, oliguria.

85. The nurse will evaluate for the most significant complication in clients undergoing chronic peritoneal dialysis, which is

1 Pulmonary embolism.

2 Hypotension.

3 Dyspnea.

4 Peritonitis.

SURGICAL QUESTIONS

86. The client who has adjusted and is well managed with intermittent hemodialysis would have a clear understanding that

1 Diet and fluid adherence between sessions will help control the development of complications.

2 His blood pressure will be adequately controlled by the hemodialysis treatments.

3 His energy level will be greatly increased following each session.

4 There will be no urine output between procedures and excess fluid will be removed during hemodialysis.

87. A 12 year old has just been returned to the unit following a tonsillectomy. A priority nursing intervention during the postoperative period is to

1 Administer oral analgesics every 4 hours.

2 Place the client in a semi-Fowler's position.

3 Apply warm compresses to the surgical site.

4 Provide cool water or apple juice to drink.

88. A client with a history of cholecystitis is now being admitted to the hospital for possible surgical intervention. The orders include NPO, IV therapy, and bedrest. In addition to assessing for nausea, vomiting and anorexia, the nurse should observe for pain

1 In the right lower quadrant.

2 After ingesting food.

3 Radiating to the left shoulder.

4 In the right upper quadrant.

89. A client scheduled for colostomy surgery will have a preoperative diet ordered that will include

1 Broiled chicken, baked potato, and wheat bread.

2 Ground hamburger, rice, and salad.

3 Broiled fish, rice, squash, and tea.

4 Steak, mashed potatoes, raw carrots, and celery.

90. The physician tells a client that he will need exploratory surgery the next day. As the RN and PN determine the preoperative teaching plan, which one of the following interventions is most important?

1 Answer questions the client has about his condition or the forthcoming surgery.

2 Explain the routine preoperative procedures: NPO, shower, medication, shave, etc.

3 Describe the surgery and what the client will experience following surgery.

4 Assure the client there is nothing to worry about because the physician is very experienced.

91. While monitoring a client's blood transfusion, the nurse determines that a hemolysis reaction is occurring. The first nursing intervention is to

   1 Slow down the transfusion.
   2 Administer IV Benadryl.
   3 Stop the transfusion.
   4 Notify the physician.

92. A client is scheduled for a kidney transplant. A medication she will probably take on a long-term basis that will require specific client teaching to ensure compliance is

   1 Corticosteroids.
   2 Antibiotics.
   3 Anticoagulants.
   4 Gamma globulin.

93. Which of the following statements is true of skeletal traction?

   1 Neurovascular complications are less apt to occur than with skin traction.
   2 The client has less mobility than he does with skin traction.
   3 Fractures can be reduced because more weight can be used than with skin traction.
   4 It is preferred for children because fracture fragment alignment is so important.

94. Russell's traction is easily recognized because it incorporates a

   1 Sling under the knee.
   2 Cervical halter.
   3 Pelvic girdle.
   4 Pearson attachment.

95. When evaluating all forms of traction, the nurse will check that the direction of pull is controlled by the

   1 Client's position.
   2 Rope/pulley system.
   3 Amount of weight.
   4 Point of friction.

96. A client scheduled for surgery is given a spinal anesthetic. Immediately following the injection, the nurse will position the client

   1 On his abdomen.
   2 In semi-Fowler's position.
   3 In slight Trendelenburg's position.
   4 On his back or side; head raised.

97. Following spinal anesthesia, a client is brought into the recovery room. During the initial data collection, which sign or symptom indicates a complication of anesthesia has developed?

   1 Hiccoughs.
   2 Numbness in legs.
   3 Headache.
   4 No urge to void.

98. A client has just arrived at the recovery room from surgery. The priority in data collection is to

   1 Assess the client's need for oxygen.
   2 Check the gag reflex.
   3 Assess vital signs.
   4 Assess airway for patency.

99. Following surgery, the client's surgeon orders a Foley catheter to be inserted. Which one of the following interventions would the nurse carry out first?

   1 Clean the perineum from front to back.
   2 Check the catheter for patency.
   3 Explain to the client that she will feel slight, temporary discomfort.
   4 Arrange the sterile items on the sterile field.

100. Assessing the client following abdominal surgery, the nurse observes pinkish fluid and a loop of bowel through an opening in the incision. The first nursing action is to

   1 Notify the physician.

2   Notify the operating room for wound closure.

3   Cover the protruding bowel with a moist, sterile, normal saline dressing.

4   Apply butterfly tapes to the incision area.

101.   A client has had a cystectomy and uretero-ileostomy (ileal conduit). The nurse observes this client for complications in the postoperative period. Which of the following symptoms indicates an unexpected outcome and requires priority care?

1   Edema of the stoma.

2   Mucus in the drainage appliance.

3   Redness of the stoma.

4   Feces in the drainage appliance.

102.   The nurse understands that it is important to obtain baseline vital signs for her client preoperatively in order to

1   Establish a baseline postoperatively.

2   Inform the anesthetist so he can administer appropriate preanesthesia medication.

3   Judge the client's recovery from the effects of surgery and anesthesia when taking postoperative vital signs.

4   Prevent operative hypotension.

103.   A client requires that a bronchoscopy procedure be done. Due to his physical condition, he will be awake during the procedure. As part of the pretest teaching, the nurse will instruct him that before the scope insertion, his neck will be positioned so that it is

1   In a flexed position.

2   In an extended position.

3   In a neutral position.

4   Hyperextended.

104.   A male, age 35, was knifed in a street fight, admitted through the emergency room, and is now in the ICU. An assessment of his condition reveals the following symptoms: respirations shallow and rapid, paradoxical pulse, CVP 15 cm H_2O, BP 90 mmHg systolic, skin cold and pale, urinary output 60–100 mL/hr for the last 2 hours. Analyzing these symptoms, the nurse will base a nursing diagnosis on the conclusion that the client has which one of the following conditions?

1   Hypovolemic shock.

2   Cardiac tamponade.

3   Wound dehiscence.

4   Atelectasis.

105.   Following an amputation, the advantage to the client for an immediate prosthesis fitting is

1   Ability to ambulate sooner.

2   Less chance of phantom limb sensation.

3   Dressing changes are not necessary.

4   Better fit of the prosthesis.

106.   Evaluating the effectiveness of preoperative teaching before colostomy surgery, the nurse expects that the client will be able to

1   Describe how the procedure will be done.

2   Exhibit acceptance of the surgery.

3   Explain the function of the colostomy.

4   Apply the colostomy bag correctly.

107.   A nursing care plan for a client with a suprapubic cystostomy would include

1   Placing a urinal bag around the tube insertion to collect the urine.

2   Clamping the tube and allowing the client to void through the urinary meatus before removing the tube.

3   Catheter irrigations every 4 hours to prevent formation of urinary stones.

4   Limiting fluid intake to 1500 mL per day.

108.   Following a treadmill test and cardiac catheterization, the client is found to have coronary artery disease which is inoperable. He is referred to the cardiac rehabilitation unit. During his first visit to the unit he says that

he doesn't understand why he needs to be there because there is nothing that can be done to make him better. The best nursing response is

1 "Cardiac rehabilitation is not a cure but can help restore you to many of your former activities."
2 "Here we teach you to gradually change your lifestyle to accommodate your heart disease."
3 "You are probably right but we can gradually increase your activities so that you can live a more active life."
4 "Do you feel that you will have to make some changes in your life now?"

109. Assessing a client who has developed atelectasis postoperatively, the nurse will be most likely to find

1 A flushed face.
2 Dyspnea and pain.
3 Decreased temperature.
4 Severe cough with no pain.

110. A client admitted to a surgical unit for possible bleeding in the cerebrum has vital signs taken every hour to monitor the neurological status. Which of the following neurological checks will give the nurse the best information about the extent of bleeding?

1 Pupillary checks.
2 Spinal tap.
3 Deep tendon reflexes.
4 Evaluation of extrapyramidal motor system.

111. Client teaching given to clients following cataract surgery should include the information that

1 The eye patch will be removed in 3 to 4 days, and the eye may be used without difficulty.
2 They must use only one eye at a time to prevent double vision.

3 They will be able to judge distances without difficulty.
4 Contact lenses will be fitted before discharge from the hospital.

112. Preoperative teaching for a client scheduled for a laryngectomy should include the fact that

1 The client will continue to be able to breathe and smell through the nose.
2 The client will be fed through a permanent gastrostomy tube.
3 The client will be able to speak again, but it will not be the same as before surgery.
4 Oral fluids will be eliminated for the first week following surgery.

113. The main complication following a nephrostomy that the nurse must assess for is

1 Bleeding from the nephrostomy site.
2 Cardiopulmonary involvement following the procedure.
3 Difficulty in restoring fluid and electrolyte balance.
4 Contamination of the site.

114. Hemorrhage is a major complication following oral surgery or radical neck dissection. If this condition occurs, the most immediate nursing intervention would be to

1 Notify the surgeon immediately.
2 Treat the client for shock.
3 Put pressure over the common carotid and jugular vessels in the neck.
4 Immediately put the client in high-Fowler's position.

115. Following laminectomy surgery, the client returns from the recovery room to the surgical unit. The nurse would anticipate that the most common complication following anesthesia would be

1 Atelectasis.
2 Pneumonia.

3   Paralytic ileus.

4   Edema.

116.   Assessing for immediate postoperative complications, the nurse knows that a complication likely to occur following unresolved atelectasis is

1   Hemorrhage.

2   Infection.

3   Pneumonia.

4   Pulmonary embolism.

117.   One method of assessing for signs of circulatory impairment in a client with a fractured femur is to ask the client to

1   Cough and deep breathe.

2   Turn himself in bed.

3   Perform biceps exercises.

4   Wiggle his toes.

118.   A 38-year-old female client is admitted to the emergency room after breaking her right wrist in a fall. Before administering the NSAID ketrololac tromethamine (Toradol) for pain, the nurse would assess for

1   Any eye problems such as glaucoma.

2   Presence of peptic ulcer disease.

3   Currently taking birth control pills.

4   An allergy to Tylenol.

119.   When a client is being instructed in crutch walking using the swing-through gait, the most appropriate directions are

1   "Look down at your feet before moving the crutches to ensure you won't fall as you move them."

2   "Place one crutch forward with the opposite foot and then place the second crutch forward followed by the second foot."

3   "Move both crutches forward then lift and swing your body past the crutches."

4   "Use the crutch bar to balance yourself to prevent falls."

120.   A cast placed on a client's leg has dried. If the drying process were completed, the nurse would observe the cast to be

1   Dull and gray in appearance.

2   Shiny and white in appearance.

3   Cool to the touch and gray in appearance.

4   Warm to the touch and white in appearance.

MEDICAL-SURGICAL NURSING

Answers with Rationale

MEDICAL ANSWERS

1. (4) Removing the tube quickly while keeping it pinched lessens the risk of gastric secretions falling into the trachea during removal. Instilling 20 to 30 mL of air, rather than normal saline, into the tube will also help prevent aspiration of gastric secretions. Unsterile gloves are worn for this procedure.

2. (3) Aqueous solutions such as Demerol readily pass through a 22 gauge needle. Larger bore needles which are more traumatizing and, therefore, more painful, are not necessary. Smaller gauge needles do not readily penetrate muscle tissue. The higher the number, the smaller the bore of the needle.

3. (1) Frequent checking and regulation of the flow is the best answer because it would include checking that the IV remains open. Recording is important, but not totally the LVN's responsibility. The IV site is changed every 48 to 72 hours.

4. (2) Aspirin can potentiate the anticoagulant effect. Analgesics without salicylates such as acetaminophen (Tylenol) should be used instead.

5. (1) An elevated blood sugar may be accompanied by ketoacidosis; therefore, it is important to test for urinary ketones when the blood glucose is over 250 mg/dL. Reducing intake may provoke hypoglycemia in a Type I diabetic. Any change in insulin dosage needs to be medically prescribed. The client should not wait 2 days before taking action when the blood sugar is high.

6. (2) Criteria for a diagnosis of AIDS in an HIV-infected person includes a CD4 lymphocyte count of less than 200.

7. (3) Milk has a high sodium content so would be restricted on a sodium restriction diet. It is necessary to check all labels for sodium content, such as perservatives. Fresh fruits and vegetables have minimal sodium content.

8. (3) The arterial oxygen supply is lowered and the demand for oxygen is increased, which results in the heart having to beat faster to meet body needs for oxygen.

9. (1) Cisplatin may depress the bone marrow, thereby interfering with the production of WBCs. The resultant leukopenia can be life-threatening; therefore, risk of infection is the highest priority. The other nursing diagnoses, although appropriate for this client, would be of lower priority.

10. (1) Depressant drugs are detoxified by the liver which is already compromised. Phenobarbital is excreted by the kidney so it is a safer medication.

11. (2) Free flow of urine together with large urine output and normal pH are antibacterial

defenses. If free flow is obstructed, the infection will most likely ascend up the tract.

12. (3) Stop or modify the bath to prevent shivering. Shivering is a method of producing body heat.

13. (2) Dicumarol is an anticoagulant drug and one of the dangers involved is bleeding. Using a safety razor can lead to bleeding through cuts. The drug should be given at the same time daily but not related to meals. Due to danger of bleeding, missed doses should not be made up.

14. (1) The drug should be given exactly on time. If the drug is given late, the client could have a myasthenic crisis and be unable to swallow the drug. If the drug is given early, the client may have a cholinergic crisis.

15. (1) Contaminated gloves should be removed without contaminating the wearer's skin (2) and (4), and without risking a tear of the gloves (3).

16. (3) Administer oxygen at 2 liters per minute and no more, for if the client is emphysemic and receives too high a level of oxygen, he will develop CO_2 narcosis and the respiratory system will cease to function.

17. (3) It is important to find out whether the drug is taken on a full or empty stomach. Gastric irritation is a common side effect of ASA therapy. It can be decreased by taking the drug with meals. An antacid can be given with the drug at bedtime; however, the nurse cannot arbitrarily tell the client to do so as it takes a physician's order.

18. (3) Diarrhea is by far the most common early sign of colchicine toxicity. When given in the acute phase of gout, the dose of colchicine is usually 0.6 mg PO q hr (not to exceed 10 tablets) until pain is relieved or gastrointestinal symptoms ensue.

19. (4) Sometimes recurrent boils are symptoms of an underlying disease process such as glycosuria. Bathing will not influence the course of the boils and they are not communicable.

20. (3) The male urethra is 6 to 8 inches long. Accepted procedure is to insert the catheter until urine begins to flow, then advance the catheter 1 to 2 inches more before attempting to inflate the balloon.

21. (4) Health professionals have the responsibility to provide clear guidelines focused on the prevention and early treatment of breast cancer. Self-examinations following menstruation coupled with annual screening examination by the physician is very effective in detecting early breast cancer.

22. (2) While all of the symptoms may be present, the characteristic problem with this condition is that of emboli. If emboli arise in the right heart chambers, they will terminate in the lungs; left chamber emboli may travel anywhere in the arterial tree.

23. (1) Carbon dioxide is insufflated into the abdomen during a laparoscopic cholecystectomy. It may irritate the diaphragm and cause referred shoulder pain. This client's complaint is a common response to this type of operation, so telling the client will be reassuring and will help to decrease the anxiety accompanying the pain.

24. (1) Periods of hyperpnea alternating with apnea is a breathing pattern that is easily missed if the client's respirations are not observed for a few minutes. It may indicate disorders of cerebral circulation, increased cerebral pressure, and/or injury to the brain tissue.

25. (1) Basilar crackles are usually heard during inspiration and are caused by sudden opening of alveoli.

26. (1) Buerger-Allen exercises improve peripheral arterial circulation and are used in the treatment of Buerger's disease. Drug therapy is the treatment of choice for Raynaud's disease; therefore, instructing about the side effects of these agents is important.

27. (3) Rheumatoid arthritis typically begins with inflammatory changes in the small joints of the hands, wrists and feet.

28. (1) High creatinine levels will be decreased. Anemia is a result of decreased production of erythropoietin by the kidney and is not affected by hemodialysis (2). Hyperkalemia and high base (bicarbonate) levels are present in renal failure clients.

29. (3) Before deflating the tracheal cuff, the nurse will apply oral or nasal suction to the airway to prevent secretions from falling into the lungs. Dressing change and humidity do not relate to suctioning.

30. (2) Whistling while exhaling prevents the bronchi from collapsing, thereby permitting more effective exhalation of trapped carbon dioxide. The other exercises do not foster exhalation of carbon dioxide.

31. (1) Lettuce contains primarily water and fiber, and is considered a "free food" in the American Dietetic Association exchange lists. The other listed foods contain significant amounts of carbohydrates and/or protein and must be computed into the diet plan.

32. (4) The most therapeutic response is to acknowledge that the client is upset and offer the opportunity to discuss these feelings. The other responses close off communication.

33. (1) Approximately 85 percent of cases of fat embolism occur within 48 hours of injury, making this the most critical time for monitoring the client for manifestations of this complication.

34. (4) A Glasgow Coma Score of 3 - 5 - 4 means that the client is able to open his eyes when spoken to and can localize pain, attempting to remove noxious stimuli when motor function is tested. He is not able to follow commands. He is able to vocalize, but is confused. Verbal response is usually tested by asking the client to state who he is, where he is, or the date.

35. (3) An unconscious person is unable to independently maintain a clear airway; therefore, the highest priority should be given to planning and providing nursing interventions that promote effective airway clearance. The other nursing diagnoses are of lower priority.

36. (2) Hypercapnia leads to vasodilation, thus increasing cerebral blood flow and increasing intracranial pressure. The client should not be encouraged to cough vigorously, as this will also raise the intracranial pressure. An intact autoregulation mechanism provides for sharp fluctuation in intracranial pressure, as might occur during coughing or sneezing in the

client without increased intracranial pressure; however, clients with increased intracranial pressure have compromised autoregulation.

37. (3) Headaches are a frequent side effect of nitroglycerin medications so giving a mild analgesic would be indicated. The nurse would not change the dose or frequency without a physician's order.

38. (2) Epidural hematomas classically present with a brief period of unconsciousness, followed by a lucid interval of varying duration, and finally followed by rapid deterioration of the level of consciousness accompanied by complaints of a severe headache.

39. (4) On dorsiflexion of the foot, the client will experience upper posterior pain in the calf if a clot is present. This is termed Homan's sign.

40. (4) Laceration, a more severe consequence of closed head injury, occurs as the brain tissue moves across the uneven base of the skull in a contusion. Contusion causes cerebral dysfunction which results in bruising of the brain. A concussion causes transient loss of consciousness, retrograde amnesia, and is generally reversible.

41. (2) Aspirin acts as an anti-inflammatory drug and, thus, reduces the inflammation of the joint. In doing so, it also relieves pain. Aspirin does not prevent extension of the disease. While aspirin reduces fever, this is not the major reason for its use in the treatment of rheumatoid arthritis.

42. (2) Food and fluids would not be given 4 to 6 hours before treatments. Because of possible problems with constipation, the foods need to be high in bulk and fiber. Small and frequent, rather than large, meals are encouraged to counter nausea and anorexia.

43. (2) Lactulose decreases blood ammonia levels in clients with hepatic coma. It is thought to decrease the colon pH through bacterial degradation.

44. (2) Decadron decreases inflammation by stabilizing leukocyte lysosomal membranes. It also suppresses the immune response so is contraindicated in clients with infection, cirrhosis and debilitating disease.

45. (4) Clients with multiple sclerosis do not usually have difficulty swallowing; therefore, techniques to promote safe swallowing would not be included on a care plan. The three other responses are important aspects in client care and should be included in the care plan.

46. (3) Hypothermia or fever may lead to an inaccurate reading. Artificial nails may distort a reading if a finger probe is used. Vasoconstriction can cause an inaccurate reading of oxygen saturation. Arterial saturations have a close correlation with the reading from the pulse oximeter as long as the arterial saturation is above 70 percent.

47. (4) The primary purposes of client education include increasing knowledge, increasing self-esteem, improving client's ability to make decisions, and facilitating behavioral changes.

48. (4) For clients with an MI, thrombolytic therapy minimizes the infarct size through lysis of the clot in the occluded coronary artery. The patent artery then promotes perfusion of the heart muscle. The other three

responses are all contraindications for the use of thrombolytic agents.

49. (1) A restrictive band 2 to 4 inches above the snake bite is most effective in containing the venom and minimizing lymphatic and superficial venous return. Elevation of the limb or immobilization would not be effective interventions.

50. (4) The word "patient" or "client" should not be used, as the chart belongs to the client; thus, adding it to the chart is redundant.

51. (4) Normal saline is the fluid of choice for irrigation. It is never advisable to force fluids into a tubing to check for patency. Sterile water and aqueous Zephiran will affect the pH of the bladder as well as cause irritation.

52. (4) The P-R interval is measured on the ECG strip from the beginning of the P wave to the beginning of the QRS complex. It is the time it takes for the impulse to travel to the ventricle.

53. (4) Pulmonary artery pressure is the most effective method of monitoring the cardiovascular system for this client. Clients with a large percentage of burned body surface often do not have an area where a cuff can be applied. Cuff blood pressures are also affected more by peripheral vascular changes. Pulse monitoring is not accurate enough to detect subtle changes in the system. Central venous pressures are less than optimal because changes in left heart pressure (sign of pulmonary edema) are often not reflected in the right heart pressures.

54. (2) Diarrhea is a very common response to the dye tablets. A dinner of tea and toast is usually given to the client. Each dye tablet is given at 5 minute intervals, usually with 1 glass of water following each tablet. The number of tablets prescribed will vary, because it is based on the weight of the client.

55. (3) The client should be taught not to do any activities or wear anything that could interfere with the free flow of blood through the arteriovenous fistula.

56. (2) Cyanosis is a result of impaired oxygen-carbon dioxide exchange at the alveolar level. Advent of the gallop (S3, S4) rhythm indicates that the client is in CHF. Cerebral/mental changes often occur but they are due to hypoxia rather than edema. Changes in the lungs occur because of increased fluid that expands in the interstitial spaces and decreased oxygen transport, not because of airway changes.

57. (1) Before moving the client, dangling at the bedside is important. This procedure stabilizes the client and allows the nurse time to assess whether he develops vertigo from a drop in blood pressure.

58. (3) An NG tube insertion is the most appropriate intervention because it will determine the presence of active gastrointestinal bleeding. A Miller-Abbott tube is a weighted, mercury-filled ballooned tube used to resolve bowel obstructions. There is no evidence of shock or fluid overload in the client; therefore, an arterial line is not appropriate at this time and an IV is optional.

59. (3) The loss should be made up over the remaining hours of the day. The nurse would not want to overhydrate the client by making up the loss too fast.

60. (3) The most important protection for the nurse is handwashing and clean gloves. She may wear a gown to protect herself if the client is not alert. A mask is advised if the client is coughing.

61. (3) A second-degree burn involves the epidermis and dermis. (1) is the definition of a fourth-degree burn, (2) is characteristic of a first-degree burn, and (4) is the definition of a third-degree burn.

62. (3) Oxygen would be ordered; however, the client should be in an orthopneic or high Fowler's position to facilitate respiratory effort. Diuretics are administered to decease circulatory overload.

63. (2) The client's instructions should include keeping the environment warm to prevent vasoconstriction. Wearing gloves, warm clothes, and socks will also be useful in preventing vasoconstriction, but TED hose would not be therapeutic. Walking will most likely increase pain.

64. (4) The presence of bile in the urine would lead to a yellow-orange or brown colored urine.

65. (4) In addition to the germicidal soap scrubs, systemic antibiotics are administered to prevent infection of the wound. Silver nitrate is not a common treatment today.

66. (2) Answer (2) is correct because the culture takes 3 weeks to grow. Usually even very small lesions can be seen on x-rays due to the natural contrast of the air in the lungs; therefore, chest x-rays do not need to be repeated frequently (3). Clients may have positive smears but negative cultures if they have been on medication (4). A positive skin test indicates the person has been infected with tuberculosis but may not necessarily have active disease (1).

67. (1) The increase in intraocular pressure causes atrophy of the retinal ganglion cells and the optic nerve, and leads eventually to blindness.

68. (3) As the liver cells become fatty and degenerate, they are no longer able to accommodate the large amount of blood necessary for homeostasis. The pressure in the liver increases and causes increased pressure in the venous system. As the portal pressure increases, fluid exudes into the abdominal cavity. This is called ascites.

69. (1) Weakness, fainting, blurred vision, pallor, and perspiration are all common symptoms when there is too much insulin or too little food—hypoglycemia. The signs and symptoms in answers (2) and (3) are indicative of hyperglycemia.

70. (3) A nursing goal is to promote physical rest and reduce stress. Discussing stressful situations may cause the client to become anxious and delay ulcer healing. Discussing the pathogenesis of ulcer disease will not help the client to relax. Identification of substances that cause pain will assist in planning for teaching. Dietary teaching should include incorporating the client's food preferences into such a regimen.

71. (1) The first specimen is discarded because it is considered "old urine" or urine that was in the bladder before the test began. After the first discarded specimen, urine is collected for 24 hours.

72. (1) It is important to decrease intracranial pressure (head of bed elevated) and to allow for drainage (head turned to left). All of the other responses are incorrect because the position would not facilitate cerebral drainage or ear drainage.

73. (3) An important assessment question is to find out how the client feels about the tests to be performed. Learning if he has talked with anyone about his concerns or fears will help the nurse assess the client's resources for emotional support and whether the client needs to talk about his fears or feelings.

74. (2) If the shunt is patent, it will feel warm to the touch and the nurse will hear the sound of rushing blood and a loud bruit. The nurse can also feel the thrill by palpating over the fistula site.

75. (2) Clients must have the head of the bed elevated to prevent the contrast medium from irritating cervical nerve roots and cranial structures. Clients may sit up in a chair following the procedure if they are comfortable.

76. (3) Clients may experience inaccurate readings if dye has been used for a diagnostic test. Dyes use colors that tint the blood which causes inaccurate readings.

77. (4) The major goal in protecting the seizure client from injury is to always maintain an adequate airway. Placing the client in a side-lying position assists in preventing aspiration. Current treatment of seizures no longer advocates the use of a padded tongue blade during a seizure because of possible injury to teeth. Restraints may also cause injury.

78. (2) Lethargy may indicate impending encephalopathy and dictate the need for client safety measures. Fatigue is expected due to anemia, shortness of breath due to ascites, and nausea due to GI vascular congestion, but these are not as grave as lethargy.

79. (4) The pain of pancreatitis is made worse by walking and supine positioning. The client is more comfortable sitting up and leaning forward.

80. (1) Frequency and dysuria are the most specific symptoms of lower urinary tract infection while (2) and (3) are more indicative of upper urinary tract infection. Cloudy urine may indicate microscopic hematuria, while odor may be related to diet.

81. (4) Infection due to catheter presence is most commonly associated with migration to the bladder along the internal lumen of the catheter after contamination. Keeping the collection bag dependent of the tubing is important to prevent reflux and contamination. The other distractors are potential, but not as common, causes of infection.

82. (4) It is most important that the client with lupus protects herself from sun exposure with large brimmed hats, long sleeves, and sunscreen cream. Keeping the skin moist and clean are also important, but lesions are best prevented by sun protection.

83. (2) Dextrose with insulin helps move potassium into cells and is immediate management therapy for hyperkalemia due to acute renal failure. An exchange resin may also be employed. This type of infusion is often administered before cardiac surgery to stabilize

irritable cells and prevent arrhythmias; in this case KCl is also added to the infusion.

84. (3) Early in progressive (chronic) renal failure, the tubules lose ability to concentrate urine so there is increased urinary output with urine of low specific gravity and concomitant increase in fluid intake. This stage goes unnoticed by most clients.

85. (4) Peritonitis is a grave complication with peritoneal dialysis. Hemodialysis may be necessary until infection clears. Excess fluid and protein effluent into the peritoneum also complicate care. Use of aseptic technique is essential.

SURGICAL ANSWERS

86. (1) It is essential that the end stage renal client adhere to all aspects of the medical regimen. Only excess solutes and fluid are removed with dialysis. Blood pressure management, aspects of care concerning concomitant anemia, and phosphate/calcium/vitamin D imbalance, as well as protein restriction and fluid restriction, must be carried out at all times. The dialysis client continues to be uremic and has multisystem problems that continue despite dialysis.

87. (4) Apple juice or water is given as soon as the client is awake and not hemorrhaging. Avoidance of citrus juices will prevent irritation of the operative site. The client should be placed on his abdomen or side to facilitate drainage and prevent aspiration. Ice bags are applied to the neck to prevent edema and bleeding.

88. (4) Pain occurs 2 to 4 hours after eating fatty foods and is located either in the epigastric re-

gion or in the upper right quadrant of the abdomen.

89. (3) The client's diet should be low residue and high calorie. Foods high in carbohydrates are usually low residue; chicken is acceptable without skin. Any salad, fresh vegetables, or grains would be considered high residue.

90. (1) It is most important to begin at the client's level of understanding, so answering questions is more essential than giving explanations until the client is ready to listen. Describing the surgery is not the nurse's responsibility, and giving false reassurance by assuring the client there is nothing to worry about is nontherapeutic.

91. (3) The first action would be to stop the transfusion to avoid administering any additional incompatible cells. The incompatible cells can lead to agglutination, oliguric renal failure, pulmonary emboli, and death if administered in large quantities. Some resources state that as little as 50 mL of incompatible blood can lead to severe complications and death.

92. (1) Prednisone, a corticosteroid, is the usual drug of choice. The other medication classifications are not used in the routine care of transplant clients.

93. (3) Because more weight can be applied with skeletal traction, it can be used to reduce fractures and maintain alignment. It is not used commonly in the elderly because of prolonged immobilization. It is not preferred for children because some displacement of fracture fragments is desirable to prevent growth disturbance. Frequently, clients have more mobility than they do with skin traction, be-

cause balanced suspension is often incorporated with skeletal traction.

94. (1) Russell's traction is a type of skin traction that incorporates a sling under the knee that is connected by a rope to an overhead bar pulley. It is frequently used to treat femoral shaft fractures in the adolescent.

95. (2) The rope/pulley and weight system is arranged so that fracture fragments are in the desired approximate position for healing. The client's position should always rest in line with the traction pull. The line of pull must never be interfered with by changing the position of a pulley and extension bar.

96. (3) Usually the client is positioned on the back following the injection. If a high level of anesthesia is desired, the head and shoulders can be lowered to slight Trendelenburg's. After 20 minutes the anesthetic is set, and the client can be positioned in any manner.

97. (3) When spinal fluid is lost through a leak or the client is dehydrated, a severe headache can occur, which may last several days. Numbness and no urge to void would be expected with spinal anesthesia unless it continues for several hours postop. The complication of hiccoughs can be associated with abdominal surgery, but is not attributable to spinal anesthesia.

98. (4) The priority assessment is to determine if the airway is patent. All of the other nursing actions will follow this assessment: need for oxygen, gag reflex and vital signs.

99. (3) It is necessary to give the client an adequate explanation for any procedure. This will result in less anxiety and more cooperation from the client.

100. (3) The first nursing action, before notifying the physician, is to cover the open wound. Evisceration will eventually have to be closed in the operating room, but this is a later step. Butterfly tapes would be applied to the wound area to prevent further dehiscence.

101. (4) The ileal conduit procedure incorporates implantation of the ureters into a portion of the ileum which has been resected from its anatomical position and now functions as a reservoir or conduit for urine. The proximal and distal ileal borders can be resumed. Feces should not be draining from the conduit. Edema and a red color of the stoma are expected outcomes in the immediate postoperative period, as is mucus from the stoma.

102. (3) It is important to have presurgery vital signs so that the client's progress can be monitored to assure that his postoperative condition is stable. A baseline is completed presurgery for evaluation postsurgery.

103. (4) Hyperextension brings the pharynx into alignment with the trachea and allows the scope to be inserted without trauma.

104. (2) All of the client's symptoms are found in both cardiac tamponade and hypovolemic shock except the increase in urinary output. In shock, urinary output decreases to less than 30 mL/hour; thus, this is the symptom that would distinguish hypovolemic shock from cardiac tamponade and form the basis for a nursing diagnosis.

105. (1)   When the prosthesis is in place immediately following surgery, the client can stand up several hours postoperatively and walk the next day. The operative site is closed to outside contamination and benefits from improved circulation due to ambulation.

106. (3)   Successful teaching can be validated when the client is able to repeat the information. A description of the surgery is irrelevant and application of the bag will be done later. Acceptance of the surgery is an emotional issue.

107. (2)   Allowing the client to void naturally will be done prior to removal of the catheter to ensure adequate emptying of the bladder. Irrigations are not recommended, as they increase the chances of the client developing a urinary tract infection. Any time a client has an indwelling catheter in place, fluids should be encouraged (unless contraindicated) to prevent stone formation.

108. (1)   Such a response does not give false hope to the client but is positive and realistic. This answer tells the client what cardiac rehabilitation is and does not dwell upon his negativity about it.

109. (2)   Atelectasis is a collapse of the alveoli due to obstruction or hypoventilation. Clients become short of breath, have a high temperature, and usually experience severe pain but do not have a severe cough. The shortness of breath is a result of decreased oxygen-carbon dioxide exchange at the alveolar level.

110. (1)   Pupillary checks reflect function of the third cranial nerve, which stretches as it becomes displaced by blood, tumor, etc.

111. (2)   The function of the lens is that of accommodation, the focusing of near objects on the retina by the lens; therefore, only the remaining lens will function in this capacity, depending on whether a cataract is present.

112. (3)   Most of the laryngectomy clients will use esophageal speech or a mechanical device for communication. They can usually begin to take oral fluids sometime after 48 hours. They are generally fed by an intravenous or nasogastric tube prior to oral feedings. Because the larynx is removed, it will be impossible to breathe through the nose.

113. (1)   While all the other conditions may be complications, bleeding from the site is the main concern. The procedure is done to achieve relief from infection caused by urinary stasis, which may have resulted in kidney congestion.

114. (3)   Putting pressure over the vessels in the neck may be life-saving because a severe blood loss can occur rapidly, leading to shock and death. The surgeon would be notified as soon as possible.

115. (1)   Even before pneumonia, atelectasis may occur as a result of the alveoli not being expanded. This leads to an alteration in gas exchange. Paralytic ileus could result from any surgery, especially if the client ingests food before the bowel is functioning properly.

116. (3)   Pneumonia is a major complication of unresolved atelectasis and must be treated along with vigorous treatment for atelectasis. Hemorrhage and infection are not related to this condition. Pulmonary embolism could result from deep vein thrombosis.

117. (4) The only activity that will indicate a complication that is directly related to impairment in circulation due to a fractured femur is the inability to wiggle his toes.

118. (2) Toradol can cause GI toxicity, ulceration or hemorrhage, especially in clients with a history of ulcers or bleeding. Salicylate levels can be increased in the serum and bleeding times can be prolonged with use of the drug.

119. (3) This is the procedure for using the swing-through gait. Clients are instructed to look straight ahead when walking with crutches. Looking down can lead to falls and uneven gait. Putting pressure from the arm on the crutch bar can cause nerve damage.

120. (2) The cast will be shiny and cool to the touch when dry. It will have a dull appearance when wet.

MATERNITY NURSING

1. In the delivery room, a client has just delivered a healthy 7-pound baby boy. The physician instructs the nurse to suction the baby. The procedure the nurse would use is to

   1 Suction the nose first.
   2 Suction the mouth first.
   3 Suction neither the nose nor mouth until the physician gives further instructions.
   4 Turn the baby on his side so mucus will drain out before suctioning.

2. The nurse is doing data collection on a post-partum client. Signs and symptoms of infection as a complication of the postpartum period would include

   1 Dark red lochia.
   2 Bradycardia.
   3 Discomfort and tenderness of the abdomen.
   4 Generalized rash.

3. A 24-year-old client who has just learned she is pregnant tells the nurse that she smokes one pack of cigarettes a day. In counseling, the nurse encourages her to stop smoking because newborns of mothers who smoke are often

   1 Premature and have respiratory distress syndrome.
   2 Small for gestational age.
   3 Large for gestational age.
   4 Born with congenital abnormalities.

4. A client, 36 weeks pregnant, is having an Oxytocin Challenge Test. After 35 minutes her uterus begins to contract, and the nurse observes three 40-second-long contractions in a 10-minute period. She has two contractions within 5 minutes, and her uterus remains con-

tracted after the second contraction. The first nursing action is to

   1 Turn off the oxytocin.
   2 Administer oxygen by mask.
   3 Turn her on her left side.
   4 Assess the fetal heart rate.

5. Oxygen and humidity are part of the treatment for premature infants. Of the following, the statement that best describes the purpose of this treatment is that it

   1 Is necessary because premature infants have a depressed Moro reflex.
   2 Facilitates perfusion of the kidney to clear blood wastes more quickly.
   3 Helps the infant adjust better to the early transition of extrauterine life.
   4 Assists the immature respiratory system with systemic oxygenation.

6. A diabetic client who is pregnant asks about breast feeding. The most accurate response regarding breast feeding by diabetic mothers is that it is

   1 Contraindicated because insulin is passed to the infant through the milk.
   2 Not contraindicated, however the diabetic's milk production and mechanism may be faulty.
   3 Contraindicated because it puts too much stress on the mother's body.
   4 Not contraindicated, but encouraged.

7. A new mother is concerned because her physician said that her baby had jaundice. The nurse understands that it is a/an

   1 Normal condition that appears at 2 to 3 days of life.

2 Normal condition that appears 8 to 24 hours after birth.

3 Abnormal condition that appears within the first 24 hours of life.

4 Abnormal condition that appears at 2 to 3 days of life.

8. A newly pregnant client who is a little overweight asks how much weight she should gain. The most appropriate answer is

1 "For your size, a little heavy, about 15 pounds would be best."

2 "It really doesn't matter exactly how much weight you gain, as long as your diet is healthy."

3 "A gain of about 25 pounds is best for mother and baby."

4 "Because you are a little overweight, it would be best for you not to gain too much weight."

9. Which one of the following statements is usually true about cervical changes in primiparas?

1 Effacement precedes dilation.

2 Effacement and dilation occur simultaneously.

3 Dilation precedes effacement.

4 Effacement is not necessary.

10. A client is 3 days postpartum. Her vital signs are stable; her fundus is 3 fingerbreadths below the umbilicus, and her lochia rubra is moderate. Her breasts are hard and warm to the touch. The nurse would conclude that the client

1 Is showing early signs of breast infection.

2 Is normal for 3 days postpartum.

3 Needs ice packs applied to her breasts.

4 Should remove her nursing bra to reduce discomfort.

11. The first day postpartum for a new mother, the nurse observes that she appears frightened and says, "The baby has been breathing funny, fast and slow, off and on." To reassure the client, a nursing response would be

1 "That's normal when the baby breast feeds."

2 "There's nothing to worry about. I'm going to take the baby back to the nursery now."

3 "I'll watch the baby for a while to see if there is something wrong."

4 "Don't be frightened. It's a normal breathing pattern. I'll sit here while you finish feeding him."

12. An amniocentesis is performed for genetic cell analysis. The nurse counsels the client that this test cannot be performed until 14 weeks gestation because

1 This is when the heartbeat is first heard.

2 The fetus is not mature enough until this time.

3 There is not enough amniotic fluid until this time.

4 The genetic results will not be accurate until this time.

13. A serology test for syphilis is given to pregnant women. The nurse explains to the client that the reason this test is given is because

1 Latent syphilis becomes highly active during pregnancy due to hormonal changes.

2 Syphilis may be passed to the fetus after 4 months of pregnancy.

3 Syphilis is no longer a problem, but the law still requires the serology test.

4 Syphilis may be passed to the infant during delivery.

14. Nursing care of a pregnant client who received regional anesthesia would include

1 Walking the client to ensure medication is evenly distributed.

2 Asking the client to turn from side to side every 15 minutes.

3 Monitoring blood pressure every 3 to 5 minutes until stabilized.

4 Giving the client sips of water to swallow during the procedure.

15. Assessing a client with eclampsia, the nurse knows that a cardinal symptom is

    1 Weight gain of 1 pound a week.
    2 Concentrated urine.
    3 Hypertension.
    4 Feeling of lassitude and fatigue.

16. The nurse would anticipate a possible complication in infants delivered by cesarean section. This condition would be

    1 Respiratory distress.
    2 Renal impairment.
    3 ABO incompatibility.
    4 Kernicterus.

17. If a client experiences a ruptured ectopic pregnancy, an expected sign or symptom would be

    1 Elevated blood glucose levels.
    2 Sudden excruciating pain in lower abdomen.
    3 Sudden hypertension.
    4 Extensive external bleeding.

18. A client, 34 weeks pregnant, has just been admitted to the labor room in the first stage of labor. Which of the following clinical manifestations would be considered abnormal and would be reported to the physician immediately?

    1 Expulsion of a blood-tinged mucous plug.
    2 Continuous contraction of 2 minutes duration.
    3 Feeling of pressure on perineum causing her to bear down.
    4 Expulsion of clear fluid from the vagina.

19. An eclamptic client has been receiving magnesium sulfate IM every 4 hours. What symptom would indicate that the next dose can safely be administered?

    1 Absence of deep tendon reflexes.
    2 A respiratory rate of 16 per minute.

    3 Urine output of 50 mL over the last 4 hours.
    4 Complaints of being thirsty.

20. An 11 lb. 6 oz. baby girl was delivered by cesarean section to a diabetic mother. The priority data collection of the infant of a diabetic mother would be for

    1 Hypoglycemia.
    2 Sepsis.
    3 Hyperglycemia.
    4 Hypercalcemia.

21. Of the following conditions, which one is not a result of metabolic error in the fetus?

    1 Phenylketonuria.
    2 Maple syrup urine disease.
    3 Glutamicacidemia.
    4 Pyloric stenosis.

22. A client has given birth to a stillborn with congenital deformities. She knows this but says she wants to see her baby. What is the nurse's best approach?

    1 "That's your right. I'll bring the baby to you."
    2 "It would be better to let your husband see the baby; then he can tell you."
    3 "Are you really sure you want to? You might regret it later."
    4 "Let's talk about it first. Tell me what you expect."

23. Of the following conditions, the one recognized as a known teratogen is

    1 Scarlet fever.
    2 Rubella.
    3 Coronary heart disease.
    4 Dental x-rays.

24. A client is gravida 3 para 2 and is in a labor room. After a vaginal exam, it is determined

that the presenting head is at station +3. The appropriate nursing action is to

1 Continue to observe the client's contractions.
2 Check the fetal heart rate for a prolapsed cord.
3 Prepare to move the client quickly to the delivery room.
4 Check with the physician to see if an oxytocin drip is warranted.

25. Pelvic inflammatory disease (PID) is an inflammatory condition of the pelvic cavity and may involve the ovaries, tubes, vascular system, or pelvic peritoneum. The nurse explains to the client that the most common cause of PID is

1 Tuberculosis bacilli.
2 Streptococcus.
3 Staphylococcus.
4 Gonorrhea.

26. Normal menstrual cycles and ovarian function are regulated by the hormones

1 FSH and LH.
2 LH and progesterone.
3 FSH and progesterone.
4 Estrogen and progesterone.

27. As the nurse walks into the newborn nursery, she sees a baby in respiratory distress from apparent mucus. The first nursing action is to

1 Carefully slap the infant's back.
2 Thump the chest and start cardiopulmonary resuscitation.
3 Pick the baby up by the feet.
4 Call the code team.

28. A client, 18 weeks pregnant, is concerned because she had a fever and rash about 2½ weeks ago. The nurse's best response is

1 "It's best to talk with the physician about that."

2 "It's unlikely the fetus would have been affected as the first trimester is the most important time."
3 "What do you think the problems are with that?"
4 "Are you thinking you may have to terminate the pregnancy?"

29. A 14 year old came to the clinic for a birth control method. She sat through the class that describes the methods available to her. After class she asked the nurse, "Which method is best for me to use?" The best response is

1 "You are so young, are you sure you are ready for the responsibilities of a sexual relationship?"
2 "Because of your age, we need your parents' consent before you can be examined and then we'll talk."
3 "Before I can help you with that question, I need to know more about your sexual activity."
4 "The physician can best help you with that after your physical examination."

30. Assessing a newborn infant, the nurse knows that postmature infants may exhibit

1 Heavy vernix, little lanugo.
2 Large size for gestational age.
3 Increased subcutaneous fat, absent creases on feet.
4 Small size for gestational age.

31. A primigravida, age 36, delivered an 8 lb. 6 oz. baby girl by cesarean section. Which one of the following nursing actions would *not* be included in the client's immediate postoperative care?

1 Taking vital signs q 15 minutes for 2 to 3 hours.
2 Checking lochia for amount and color q 15 minutes for 2 to 3 hours.
3 Assisting the client to turn, cough and deep breathe.
4 Offering oral fluids q 15 minutes for 2 to 3 hours.

32. Counseling a client who is starting to use oral contraception, the nurse explains that birth control pills work by the mechanism of

   1 Inhibiting chorionic gonadotropin production.
   2 Inhibiting follicle-stimulating hormone production.
   3 Inhibiting progesterone and estrogen production.
   4 Stimulating luteinizing hormone production.

33. Which of the following garments worn by a pregnant woman would necessitate a special nursing intervention?

   1 Garter belt with nylon stockings.
   2 Support panty hose.
   3 Woolen athletic socks.
   4 Knee-high nylon sockettes.

34. An appropriate nursing intervention to help a nursing mother care for cracked nipples would be

   1 Applying benzoin to toughen the nipples.
   2 Keeping the nipples covered with warm, moist packs.
   3 Offering to give the baby a bottle.
   4 Exposing the nipples to air as much as possible.

35. A client is very concerned because her 1-day-old son, who was very alert at birth, is now sleeping most of the time. The appropriate nursing response would be

   1 "Most infants are alert at birth and then require 24 to 48 hours of deep sleep to recover from the birth experience."
   2 "Your son's behavior is slightly abnormal and bears careful observation."
   3 "Would you like the pediatrician to check him to ease your mind?"
   4 "Your son's behavior is definitely abnormal, and we should keep him in the nursery."

36. During a physical exam of an infant with congenital hip dysplasia, the nurse would notice which of the following characteristics?

   1 Symmetrical gluteal folds.
   2 Limited adduction of the affected leg.
   3 Palpable femoral pulse when the hip is flexed and the leg is abducted.
   4 Limited abduction of the affected leg.

37. A neonatal nurse would be aware that small-for-gestational age infants (SGA) are more likely to develop which of the following neonatal illnesses?

   1 Hyperthermia.
   2 Hyperglycemia.
   3 Congenital defects.
   4 Hypothermia.

38. If RhoGAM is given to a mother after delivering a healthy baby, the condition that must be present for the globulin to be effective is that the

   1 Mother is Rh positive.
   2 Baby is Rh negative.
   3 Mother has no titer in her blood.
   4 Mother has some titer in her blood.

39. A client delivered a 34-week, 1550-gm female infant. The infant demonstrates nasal flaring, intercostal retraction, expiratory grunt, and slight cyanosis. The baby will be placed in a heated isolette because

   1 The infant has a small body surface for her weight.
   2 Heat increases flow of oxygen to extremities.
   3 Her temperature control mechanism is immature.
   4 Heat within the isolette facilitates drainage of mucus.

40. A 28-year-old client has just learned that her pregnancy test is positive. The nurse will rein-

force nutritional counseling by telling the client that her diet should

1 Maintain iron intake and increase calorie intake by 500 calories.
2 Increase iron and increase calorie intake by 300 calories.
3 Increase iron and multivitamins but maintain calorie intake.
4 Decrease iron but increase calorie intake by 200 to 300 calories.

MATERNITY NURSING

Answers with Rationale

1. (2) It is important to suction the mouth first. If the nose were to be suctioned first, stimulation of the delicate receptors in the nose could cause the infant to aspirate mucus from the mouth.

2. (3) The major symptoms of infection would be rapid pulse, foul-smelling lochia or discharge, and discomfort and tenderness of the abdomen. A generalized rash would not be a sign of postpartum infection but would indicate a virus infection, such as measles, or an allergic reaction to a medication or food. A rash should never be ignored; rather it should be charted and its cause investigated.

3. (2) Women who smoke have almost twice the chance of delivering a low-birth weight infant (less than 2500 grams) than nonsmokers.

4. (1) The first action is to turn the Pitocin off. If the fetal heart rate has dropped in response to the prolonged contraction, turning the mother on her side and administering oxygen may be necessary.

5. (4) The premature infant's poorly developed ability to control respirations is a frequent problem. Additional respiratory support with oxygen will decrease potential hypoxemia. The oxygen will also help oxygenate the systemic circulation if the infant has a tendency for hypoventilation.

6. (4) Insulin does not cross into the milk. The mother's calorie intake needs to be adjusted with increased protein intake. Insulin must be adjusted and care must be exercised during weaning. Breast feeding may actually have an antidiabetogenic effect and this requires less insulin.

7. (1) Jaundice (icterus neonatorum) is a normal newborn condition that appears 48 to 72 hours after birth and begins to subside on the sixth to seventh day. If the levels go above 13 mg per 100 mL, it is considered to be beyond the "safe" physiologic limit. The condition is caused by the breakdown of excess fetal red blood cells after birth.

8. (3) The optimum weight gain for both mother's and baby's health is about 25 pounds. Dieting is contraindicated. There is a lower incidence of prematurity, stillbirths, and low birth-weight infants with a weight gain of at least 25 pounds.

9. (1) Primiparas normally go through effacement before dilation of the cervix. Multiparas tend to dilate and efface simultaneously.

10. (2) From the assessment findings of the lochia and fundus, the new mother is progressing normally during the postpartum period. The breast signs indicate normal engorgement which occurs about 3 days after birth. With stable vital signs, infection is not likely to be a problem. Applying warm packs and wearing a nursing bra will reduce discomfort.

11. (4) An infant's normal breathing pattern is irregular. Staying with the client helps give her support, and the nurse can reassure her that the infant is all right.

12. (3) Amniocentesis cannot be done until adequate amniotic fluid is available, which is at about 14 weeks gestation. It usually is done for genetic counseling purposes before 18 weeks, as the test result requires 2 to 4 weeks, and elective abortion after 22 weeks is contraindicated. Chorionic Villus Sampling (CVS) may replace this test as diagnostic information is available from 8 to 12 weeks.

13. (2) The venereal disease syphilis is again becoming increasingly prevalent. It may cause abortion early in pregnancy and may be passed to the fetus after the fourth month of pregnancy, causing congenital syphilis in the infant. Gonorrhea and herpes virus II may be passed to the infant during delivery, but syphilis is usually passed to the infant in utero.

14. (3) Regional anesthesia, such as a caudal or epidural, may result in vasodilatation by causing blood to pool in the extremities. This may lead to maternal hypotension so the BP should be monitored. Immediate treatment is to elevate both legs for a few minutes in order to return the blood to the central circulation and then turn the client on her side to reduce pressure on the veins and arteries in the pelvic area.

15. (3) High blood pressure is one of the cardinal symptoms of toxemia or eclampsia along with excessive weight gain, edema and albumin in the urine.

16. (1) During a normal birth, the fetus passes through the birth canal and pressure on the chest helps rid the fetus of amniotic fluid that has accumulated in the lungs. The baby delivered by cesarean section does not go through this process, and thus, may develop respiratory problems.

17. (2) In a ruptured ectopic pregnancy, there may be signs of shock, excruciating pain, and minimal bleeding. There should be no effect on blood glucose levels.

18. (2) A uterus that is contracted for more than 1 full minute is a sign of tetany which could lead to uterine rupture. This symptom must be reported to the physician immediately so interventions can be initiated. The other answers are all normal conditions which occur with labor. The client should be cautioned against bearing down this early as it is not effective and can cause edema of the cervix.

19. (2) The respiratory rate must be maintained at a rate of at least 12 per minute as a precaution against excessive depression of impulses at the myoneural junction. When deep tendon reflexes are absent and the urine output is decreased, the medication should be held to prevent complications of depression of the CNS. If the client is complaining of being thirsty, she is experiencing a sign of magnesium toxicity.

20. (1) Infants of diabetic mothers are prone to develop hypoglycemia, respiratory distress, and hypocalcemia. The infant of a diabetic mother may develop sepsis, but usually from a cause unrelated to the diabetes itself. Hyperbilirubinemia is also fairly common in these infants.

21. (4) This is an example of a congenital abnormality and does not fall into the category of a

metabolic or biochemical disorder. Phenylketonuria is an inability to metabolize the amino acid, phenylalanine; maple syrup urine disease is defective metabolism of branched chain keto acids; glutamicacidemia is an increase in total amino nitrogen.

22. (4) The mother has a right to see her infant, but must have some anticipatory guidance. Finding out what the mother's expectations are will help the nurse better prepare the mother to see her dead child.

23. (2) *Teratogen* is a term denoting "monster-former," and rubella in the first trimester is known to produce monster babies. X-rays are also considered teratogens. Dental x-rays would not have high roentgens, thus they have little chance of being dangerous.

24. (3) If the head is +3, it is just about crowning, and because the client is a multipara, it would be reasonable to assume delivery is imminent. Answers (1) and (4) are not appropriate nursing actions and answer (2) is wrong because there is no data suggesting a prolapsed cord.

25. (4) Gonorrhea accounts for 65 to 75 percent of all cases of PID. Streptococcus, staphylococcus, and Tb bacilli are less frequent causes.

26. (1) Normal menstrual cycles and ovarian function are regulated by FSH and LH, which are produced in the hypothalamus.

27. (3) The airway must be cleared before anything else can help. Of the choices, (3) is the best for clearing the airway by creating a gravity or postural drainage situation.

28. (3) Although the first trimester is the danger period with German measles, the nurse should first ascertain the client's concerns before she gives any direction. Answer (4) is putting words in the client's mouth.

29. (3) Consultation with a client on the best form of birth control for her is dependent on the frequency of intercourse, number of partners, and her own motivation and reliability. The other responses cut off the client and do not form a therapeutic relationship.

30. (4) Babies that are postmature often look as though they have lost weight. They exhibit long nails, little subcutaneous fat, and the skin is very dry. Often, meconium is stained green or yellow.

31. (4) Oral fluids are usually withheld after surgery until normal conscious levels are reached and bowel sounds are heard. Giving oral fluids before normal consciousness returns can lead to vomiting and aspiration. A C-section is also considered a surgical procedure, and normal postop as well as postpartum care should be given.

32. (2) Birth control pills are small doses of estrogen and progesterone that maintain sufficient levels in the body to inhibit the pituitary from producing the follicle-stimulating hormone.

33. (4) These stockings are held up by elastic bands around the leg and may cause constriction of blood vessels. Frequently, women are more susceptible to varicose veins, and this would aggravate the problem. Any tightly constrictive clothing on the legs should be avoided by everyone, and especially by pregnant women.

34. (4) Keeping the nipples dry is the best treatment. Massé cream or pure lanolin may be applied sparingly, but never harsh agents such as benzoin or alcohol. Teach the mother to use general hygiene practices—wash the breasts once daily; do not use soap as it removes natural oils. To prevent further problems with engorgement, bottles should not be offered.

35. (1) Normally most newborns are alert at birth and then require deep sleep to recover from the birth experience. This should be explained first, and then if the client is still concerned, the nurse could offer to have the pediatrician talk to her.

36. (4) Abduction is limited in the affected leg. The nurse would also find asymmetrical gluteal folds and an absent femoral pulse when the affected leg is abducted.

37. (4) A large proportion of body surface to body weight increases susceptibility to hypothermia. These infants are also more prone to hypoglycemia. Congenital defects are not neonatal illnesses.

38. (3) RhoGAM will not work if there is any titer in the blood; thus it is important to administer it within 72 hours after delivery or abortion if the mother shows no evidence of antibody production. The mother would be Rh negative and the baby Rh positive for RhoGAM to be needed.

39. (3) The premature infant has poor body control of temperature and needs immediate attention to keep from losing heat. Reasons for heat loss include little subcutaneous fat and poor insulation, large body surface for weight, immaturity of temperature control, and lack of activity.

40. (2) During pregnancy iron supplements must be added to the diet because studies have found that pregnant women cannot assimilate enough iron from their regular diet. Calories are increased by 300 to be certain that the mother-to-be and fetus have enough nutritional intake.

PEDIATRIC NURSING

1. The nurse is caring for a hospitalized toddler who was toilet trained at home. He wets his pants. The best response to this situation is to say

   1. "It's okay; try not to wet your pants next time."
   2. "That's okay; now let's get you cleaned up."
   3. "I know you understand how to use the toilet; what happened?"
   4. "Your mom told me you don't wet anymore; what's wrong?"

2. The nurse is completing a general assessment on a neonate. The nurse will suspect Hirschsprung's disease when the neonate

   1. Has foul smelling, ribbonlike stools and is anemic.
   2. Fails to pass meconium within 24 to 48 hours after birth and is reluctant to ingest fluids.
   3. Is continuously hungry and fails to gain weight.
   4. Has 7 to 8 watery, bile-containing stools in the first 24 to 48 hours after birth.

3. A mother calls the pediatric hotline and tells the nurse that her 3 year old has a virus and a fever. She asks how much aspirin she should give the child. The best response is

   1. "You'll have to call your physician."
   2. "Give her no more than 3 baby aspirin every 4 hours."
   3. "Give her Tylenol, not aspirin."
   4. "Follow directions on the aspirin bottle for her age and weight."

4. An infant was born with spina bifida and has remained on the pediatric unit for observa-

   tion. The most important assessment would be to

   1. Measure head circumference daily.
   2. Monitor for contractures.
   3. Observe for signs of infection.
   4. Observe intake and output.

5. The nurse will provide teaching to the parents of infants with gastroesophageal reflux. Included in these instructions will be directions to

   1. Feed the baby only when the baby is hungry.
   2. Maintain the desired positioning and adhere to a frequent feeding schedule.
   3. Allow the baby to complete the feeding before attempting to burp the baby.
   4. Place the baby in a supine position with the head of the bed elevated at least 45 degrees.

6. Which one of the following characteristics of acute glomerulonephritis is it essential for the nurse to know in order to deliver comprehensive care to a 5-year-old child?

   1. Polyuria (increased urine output) is a clinical manifestation of this disorder.
   2. Acute glomerulonephritis is usually preceded by a streptococcal infection of the upper respiratory tract or skin.
   3. It is necessary to monitor for hypotension and tachycardia.
   4. Weight loss is a common clinical manifestation.

7. The best place to check the pulse of an infant is at the

   1. Carotid artery.
   2. Apex of the heart.

3 Brachial artery.

4 Temporal artery.

8. Proper depth of compressions for infant (under 12 months) CPR would be

1 ½ to 1 inch.

2 ¼ to ¾ inch.

3 1 to 1½ inches.

4 1½ to 2 inches.

9. A systolic blood pressure of 60 mmHg or less would indicate shock in which of the following client age groups?

1 5 years old or younger.

2 5 to 12 years old.

3 12 to 16 years old.

4 16 to 20 years old.

10. When assessing a child with hydrocephalus who has a ventriculoperitoneal (VP) shunt, the nurse would be most concerned about a recent

1 Growth spurt, increased appetite, and thirst.

2 Upper respiratory infection with coughing, a recent growth spurt, and a palpable shunt catheter.

3 Growth spurt, fever, and irritability changing to lethargy.

4 Diarrhea, recent weight loss, and a soft, round abdomen.

11. When providing diversional activities for a child in isolation, the nurse will remember that

1 Any articles brought into the unit should be washable.

2 These children are always on bedrest.

3 The room is usually darkened to protect the child's eyes.

4 Most children are satisfied with books.

12. In children, the period of negativism begins when the child

1 Can manipulate his or her parents.

2 Copies negative behavior of siblings.

3 Is struggling between dependence and independence.

4 Is learning manual skills.

13. Which of the following procedures is contraindicated in infantile eczema?

1 Have the child vaccinated to prevent childhood diseases.

2 Cover the child's hands and feet with cotton materials.

3 Apply open wet dressings or corn starch.

4 Adhere strictly to an elimination diet.

14. A child has been admitted to the pediatric unit with the diagnosis of congestive heart failure (CHF). The nurse knows that *early* symptoms of CHF include

1 Arrhythmias and conduction blocks.

2 Hypotension, decreased urine output, and weak pedal pulses.

3 Cyanosis, peripheral edema, and bradycardia.

4 Hepatomegaly, bulging fontanelles, and tachypnea.

15. Considering a 17-month-old child's developmental level, the most effective technique to reestablish nutritional status after the immediate postoperative period would be

1 Semisoft foods QID.

2 Finger foods at frequent intervals.

3 Regular diet put into a blender and given in liquid state.

4 A high-roughage diet.

16. A 2-year-old toddler was diagnosed with iron-deficiency anemia. Which one of the following statements best describes the anemias of childhood?

1   The clinical manifestations of anemia are directly related to the decrease in oxygen-carrying capacity of the blood.
2   Significant deficiencies of all vitamins will result in reduced production of red blood cells.
3   A 2-year-old child with a hemoglobin of 5 gm/100 mL will not manifest signs and symptoms of the disorder.
4   All anemias in childhood are potentially terminal.

17.   The nurse has just completed data collection for a 4-year-old child. Which one of the following findings is most characteristic of thrombocytopenia?

1   Petechiae, hematuria, purpura.
2   Urticaria, epistaxis, hypertension.
3   Purpura, tachycardia, hypotension.
4   Vertigo, petechiae, bradycardia.

18.   When determining if a child has Down's syndrome characteristics, which of the following would *not* be present?

1   Abnormal palmar creases.
2   Protruding tongue.
3   Low-set ears.
4   Loose joints and flaccid muscles.

19.   When assessing clinical indicators of adequate cardiac output in children, which of the following signs are *most* important?

1   Blood pressure, skin temperature, and capillary refill.
2   Pedal pulses, blood pressure, and skin temperature.
3   Pedal pulses, skin temperature, and capillary refill.
4   Blood pressure, urine output, and skin temperature.

20.   A mother with a 4-month-old infant comes to the clinic for a well-baby examination. The nurse advises the mother to change the formula she is feeding the baby to one that con-

tains iron. The nurse explains the reason for this is

1   Iron is required by the infant's eyes as they begin to focus and develop.
2   The infant requires extra iron to grow.
3   The infant's iron source from the mother is depleted.
4   The infant requires more iron for the breakdown of bilirubin.

21.   A 1-month-old child manifests all of the following signs and symptoms. Which of these is most suggestive of a complication of a central nervous system infection?

1   Separation of cranial sutures.
2   Depressed anterior fontanel.
3   Oliguria.
4   Photophobia.

22.   A child with the diagnosis of Guillain-Barré Syndrome would have which of the following nursing diagnoses included on the care plan?

1   Fluid Volume Deficit; Impaired Gas Exchange; and Altered Nutrition.
2   Ineffective Breathing Pattern; Pain; and Urinary Incontinence.
3   Urinary Incontinence; High Risk for Impaired Skin Integrity; and Ineffective Airway Clearance.
4   Impaired Gas Exchange; Anticipatory Grieving; and Pain.

23.   An obese 14 year old is admitted to the adolescent unit with a tentative diagnosis of type I diabetes mellitus. Adolescent diabetics frequently have more difficulty than diabetics in other age groups because

1   The disease is usually more severe in adolescents than in younger children.
2   Adolescents as a group have poor eating habits.
3   Adolescents have a difficult time with long-acting insulin.
4   Adolescents have difficulty regulating their insulin.

24. A first-grader was sent to the school nurse by her teacher because the teacher feared the child had lice in her hair. The most effective way of recognizing lice instead of dandruff is to know that

   1 Prepubescent children rarely have dandruff.
   2 There will be an area of alopecia on the nape of her neck.
   3 The child is scratching her head almost incessantly.
   4 Lice would not fall off the hair shaft when the hair is moved.

25. What anatomical condition must be present in order for an infant with complete transposition of the great vessels to survive at birth?

   1 Coarctation of the aorta.
   2 Large septal defect.
   3 Pulmonic stenosis.
   4 Mitral stenosis.

26. When taking the history from the mother of a baby who has pyloric stenosis, the nurse would expect her to say that the baby vomits

   1 Continuously.
   2 Immediately after feedings.
   3 Between feedings.
   4 When new foods are introduced.

27. A child with hemophilia A has experienced an episode of hemarthrosis. The most appropriate intervention to implement is to

   1 Teach the parents to offer aspirin for comfort.
   2 Apply an ice pack.
   3 Encourage ambulation.
   4 Apply pressure for at least 5 minutes.

28. The diet regimen the nurse will follow for a child with acute glomerulonephritis is

   1 Low sodium, low calorie.
   2 Low potassium, low protein.

   3 Fluid intake of 1000 mL/24 hours.
   4 Low calcium, low potassium.

29. Assessing a child with a possible cardiac condition, the nurse knows that a child with a large patent ductus arteriosus would exhibit which of the following symptoms?

   1 Often assuming a squatting position.
   2 Becomes cyanotic on exertion.
   3 Is acyanotic but has difficulty breathing after physical activity.
   4 Has breathing difficulty and is cyanotic with slight activity.

30. The best position for an infant with extrophy of the bladder is

   1 Prone.
   2 Supine, flat.
   3 Sidelying.
   4 Trendelenburg's.

31. A young client with cystic fibrosis is receiving dornase-alfa (Pulmozyme). To check for the desired therapeutic effect, the nurse would monitor the client's

   1 Weight.
   2 Lung sounds.
   3 Cardiac rhythm.
   4 Serum chloride.

32. Which one of the following therapeutic approaches would be appropriate in the nursing/medical management of a 12 year old with juvenile rheumatoid arthritis?

   1 Encourage prolonged periods of complete joint immobilization.
   2 Apply warm compresses and night splints to the affected joint.
   3 Discourage the child's active participation in his care in the initial phases of the disease.
   4 Allow unlimited salicylates as necessary for control of pain.

33. A client gave birth to a baby who weighed only 5 pounds and is considered premature. One of the most important principles in providing nutrition is to

    1 Use a regular nipple with a large hole.
    2 Feed every 4 to 6 hours.
    3 Use a premie nipple for bottle feeding.
    4 Use milk high in fat for the formula.

34. A child is admitted with the diagnosis of cystic fibrosis. The nurse would observe for pulmonary complications that would present as

    1 Coughing paroxysms that are worse at night.
    2 Hyperinflation with copious, thin, clear secretions at the alveolar level.
    3 Local consolidation on chest x-ray and a decreased AP diameter.
    4 A diffuse pattern of bronchial and bronchiolar obstruction with secondary infections.

35. To obtain an apical pulse on an infant, the diaphragm of the stethoscope is placed at the apex of the heart. When placing the diaphragm on the infant's chest, it should be located

    1 At the left nipple, where the heart's point of maximum impulse is located.
    2 To the left of the midclavicular line, at the third to fourth intercostal space.
    3 At the left edge of the sternum and fifth intercostal space.
    4 At the left midclavicular line and fifth intercostal space.

36. A 10-year-old child in respiratory difficulty is admitted to the emergency room and given epinephrine with oxygen ordered PRN. The nurse observes that he is short of breath with circumoral cyanosis and sweating. The nursing action will be to

    1 Notify the physician immediately.
    2 Encourage the child to lie down and administer oxygen.

    3 Reassure the child that the medication will begin working soon.
    4 Encourage the child to sit upright and administer oxygen.

37. Once a child has had one poison ingestion, statistically he is nine times more likely to have another poisoning episode within the year. To prevent further poisoning incidents, the most important information the nurse should give to the child's mother is to

    1 Keep purses out of the child's reach.
    2 Never give medications to others in front of the child.
    3 Keep all cabinets locked at all times.
    4 Keep medicine only in high cupboards.

38. An infant warmer is used in the newborn nursery to ensure maintenance of adequate body temperature. The major safety factor involved with the use of the warmer is for the nurse to

    1 Ensure the warmer is on manual control.
    2 Tape the thermometer skin probe in place.
    3 Inspect the skin under the temperature probe at routine intervals.
    4 Adjust temperature of the warmer each day to ensure it is set at 102° F.

39. Working with children who have acyanotic heart defects, the nurse is aware that

    1 Occurrence of cardiac failure is rare after the age of 6 months.
    2 Bacterial endocarditis is not a complication of acyanotic congenital heart disease.
    3 An infant or young child with acyanotic heart disease requires alteration in their activity level by their parents.
    4 Children with congenital heart disease are usually asymptomatic.

40. The nurse explains to the mother of a 1 year old that the child is more likely to have otitis media than her 13-year-old brother because

1 Her hands are often contaminated when she crawls on the floor.
2 She is still "cutting" new teeth.
3 The angle of the child's eustachian tube is straighter than her brother's.
4 She is not old enough to have learned how to "clear" her nasal passages.

41. With a diagnosis of hemophilia B, part of the teaching plan for a child's parents will include treatment measures to control minor bleeding episodes. These will include

1 Topical coagulants, cold packs, and constant pressure to affected areas.
2 Elevation of the affected area, oral anticoagulants, and warm compresses.
3 Gentian violet, ice packs, and pressure dressings.
4 Bedrest, topical coagulants, and cold compresses.

42. A mother of a 3-month-old infant asks the nurse if her baby can eat solid food now so she can sleep through the night. The appropriate response is to say

1 "Infants obtain all the nutrients they need from the formula and they really can't digest foods well at that early age."
2 "Infants at age 3 months do not usually sleep through the night, so solid food probably will not help this problem."
3 "It would be best to give the baby her bath at night to relax her and then she might sleep through the night."
4 "It sounds like she's not getting enough food to satisfy her, so it is probably a good idea to start introducing solid food."

43. While a 1 year old is hospitalized with bronchitis, she is receiving care for the respiratory condition. An appropriate toy for her would be a

1 Book with pop-up pages.
2 Set of blocks.
3 Mobile hanging from the crib.
4 Terry cloth teddy bear.

44. A 2-year old has been admitted to the pediatric unit for a diagnostic workup. When his mother left, the child cried, screamed and threw toys out of his bed. The nurse will recognize this behavior as

1 A spoiled child.
2 A sign of mental retardation.
3 Separation anxiety.
4 Normal.

45. An appropriate nursing intervention when caring for an infant with an acute upper respiratory infection and elevated temperature would be to

1 Give frequent cold sponge baths to decrease the fever.
2 Push solid food intake to maintain caloric needs.
3 Give small amounts of clear liquids frequently to prevent dehydration.
4 Dress the child warmly to prevent chilling.

PEDIATRIC NURSING

Answers with Rationale

1. (2) The nurse knows that children tend to regress when under the stress of hospitalization, so it is important not to make a judgment or imply that the child should know better. The best approach: be matter-of-fact, not blaming.

2. (2) These are signs of decreased autonomic innervation to the colon, classic Hirschsprung's Disease. The other answers indicate other intestinal disorders.

3. (3) Children from 2 months to adolescence are advised not to take aspirin with a virus infection due to the connection to Reye's Syndrome, an acute encephalopathy condition. Tylenol is the treatment of choice for any virus infection.

4. (1) While all of the assessments would be done, the most important is to measure head circumference daily. An increase in size would indicate a neurological condition developing (hydrocephalus is a frequent complication). Infection might occur in the urinary tract; I & O is also related to the possible urological complications. Contractures could be prevented through proper positioning.

5. (2) Positioning will decrease the amount of reflux and consistent feeding schedules will decrease the tendency to overfeed if the child is very hungry. Small meals tend to cause less reflux.

6. (2) This is important to understand because antibiotics are one of the primary aspects of care if the disorder was preceded by an infection of group-A beta-hemolytic streptococci. (1) is wrong because there is decreased urine output with edema formation. Answer (3) is a complication.

7. (3) The brachial artery should be used in checking the pulse of an infant. Apical pulse observation may give incomplete data because there is not adequate blood circulation. The carotid arteries are difficult to locate in an infant.

8. (1) The proper depth of compression for infant CPR is ½ to 1 inch. This is done midsternum, using only two fingers or the thumbs, if the chest is encircled by the rescuer's hands.

9. (2) A systolic blood pressure of 60 mmHg or less found in children 5 to 12 years old would indicate shock.

10. (3) The major complication of VP shunts are infection and malfunction. Children can "outgrow" shunts or distal ends can dislodge after growth spurts. Fever can be a sign of an infected shunt, and irritability deteriorating to lethargy could be due to increased intracranial pressure (ICP) from a blocked shunt. Appetite usually decreases with increasing ICP; respiratory infections should not change shunt patency.

11. (1) Things that go into the room will have to be disinfected before they are removed, so they should be washable. The children are not always on bedrest, nor does the room necessarily have to be dark.

12. (3) Negativism begins as the child learns to do some things independently and then becomes frustrated by things he or she cannot do. This period begins at about 2 years and is normal for this stage of development.

13. (1) The vaccine can cause vaccinia, which can superimpose the pustular eruptions of the viral infection on the eczema. Eliminating foods that exacerbate the problem is helpful, but not using any specific diet. Applying soaks with Burow's solution or normal saline is the treatment of choice.

14. (4) A child's liver becomes engorged early on in CHF and hepatomegaly is easily palpated. Bulging fontanels and tachypnea are signs of fluid overload. Arrhythmias and conduction changes may occur later in response to hypoxia; cyanosis, hypotension and decreased urine output are *late* signs.

15. (2) The developmental period is the autonomy stage. The child wants to do things for himself and will respond well to finger foods offered frequently. If the child will eat a variety of nutritious finger foods, the nutritional status will be reestablished more effectively.

16. (1) Clinical manifestations of fatigability, anorexia, weakness, and tachycardia are a result of vitamin B_{12} and folic acid deficiency. This results in reduced production of red blood cells, and a 2-year-old child will manifest symptoms of this disorder.

17. (1) Thrombocytopenia (a platelet count 50,000 or below) is characterized by petechiae, purpura and, on occasion, spontaneous hematuria. The lower the platelet count, the greater the risk of spontaneous bleeding.

18. (3) Although low-set ears are a sign of congenital defects, they are usually associated with some kidney problem. The other characteristics will be present with Down's syndrome.

19. (3) Children can maintain normal blood pressure when experiencing serious hemodynamic deficits. Signs of peripheral perfusion change early in assessing decreased cardiac output and are reliable clinical indicators. Urine output is a late sign.

20. (3) Between 3 and 5 months, the infant has used up the iron provided by the mother and requires further supplementation if bottle feeding.

21. (1) Meningitis is a common CNS infection of infancy and early childhood. Increased intracranial pressure, which can accompany meningitis, accounts for separation of the cranial sutures, bulging fontanels, and/or projectile vomiting. Oliguria and photophobia are not symptoms common to CNS infection.

22. (3) As paralysis progresses, urinary incontinence becomes a problem; skin can break down without frequent positioning changes and exercises. Airway problems are of major concern with ascending paralysis. Pain is generally not a problem, nor is gas exchange unless the airway is compromised and lung function affected by chest paralysis.

23. (2) As young adults start spending more time with their peer group, they frequently adopt eating habits of this group which are often not appropriate for diabetics.

24. (4) Lice secrete a cementlike substance which allows them to hold tenaciously onto the hair shaft. Dandruff will easily brush off. Alopecia, loss of hair, will not occur.

25. (2) Because complete transposition results in two closed blood systems, the child can survive only if a large septal defect is present.

26. (2) Stenosis of the pyloric sphincter impedes gastric emptying; therefore, feedings are vomited when the stomach is full.

27. (2) Ice will produce vasoconstriction to help control bleeding into the joint and promote comfort. Aspirin and ambulation will provoke further bleeding. Pressure to the joints is ineffective in controlling internal bleeding.

28. (2) A diet restricted from potassium and protein is necessary for all children who demonstrate some degree of renal failure. For severe renal failure, protein is totally restricted.

29. (3) PDA is acyanotic. If the ductus is large and much blood is shunted into the pulmonary circulation, there may be growth retardation and limitation of physical activity. Squatting occurs with cyanotic disorders.

30. (3) Placing an infant in a sidelying position will promote the drainage of urine from the bladder and help reduce the risk of urinary tract infection.

31. (2) Dornase-alfa reduces the viscosity of the sputum in clients with cystic fibrosis. Pulmonary function is improved and the incidence of respiratory tract infections is lessened. Lung sounds reflect the presence or absence of lung congestion which may indicate infection and are, therefore, monitored closely as an indicator of the therapeutic effect of this drug.

32. (2) Warm compresses will help to relieve the pain and night splints are important. During an exacerbation of this childhood disorder, hospitalization is usually required; however, affected joints should *not* be immobilized for extended periods of time as residual effects (joint atrophy) will ensue. Active participation in care should be encouraged in all stages of the disease. Unlimited salicylates could be dangerous to the child.

33. (3) A regular nipple is too hard and will make it difficult for the infant to suck, causing unnecessary fatigue. Use a premie soft nipple.

34. (4) Mechanical obstruction from thick, tenacious secretions is a major problem, causing bronchiolar obstruction and a pattern of infections. Air trapping and wheezing occur with increased AP diameter of the chest. Nocturnal coughing paroxysms may occur more commonly with pertussis.

35. (2) This is the appropriate location on an infant's chest for an apical pulse. Over age 7, the apical pulse is found at the location described in answer (4).

36. (4) The child's immediate situation needs to be addressed before calling the physician. Epinephrine is usually effective immediately.

Breathing is more effective in an upright position; oxygen is indicated from the symptoms.

37. (3) The other answers are also necessary information but keeping cabinets locked is critical. It is not enough to keep only medicine in high cupboards because other products, such as cleaning materials, can be poison. The child's mother should also be given the telephone number of a poison control center.

38. (3) The probe can cause irritation. If this occurs, the probe is placed in a different location. An infant's skin is very delicate and becomes irritated easily.

39. (1) Cardiac failure rarely occurs after the age of 6 months. If the child has gone 6 months without failure, then either the cardiac problem is not severe or the child is compensating successfully. Bacterial endocarditis is a possible complication (2) and usually a child sets his own pace of activity (3).

40. (3) It is easier for infectious agents to travel from the nasopharyngeal area to the middle ear in younger than in older children because the eustachian tube is straighter when they are younger.

41. (1) Local measures which sometimes help control minor bleeding episodes are topical coagulants, constant pressure, and cold packs (which cause vasoconstriction) to the bleeding areas.

42. (1) Studies have indicated that breast milk or formula will provide sufficient nutrition to infants up to 6 months and even 1 year. Many pediatricians begin introducing solid food about 6 months of age, because infants cannot easily digest food before this time. Sleeping patterns for infants vary on an individual basis and the introduction of solid food does not ensure a full night's sleep.

43. (4) Because the child is in a mist tent, she will need a toy that can get wet, then dry out. A book (1) might not last in this misty environment. The blocks (2) would be difficult to play with and the mobile (3) is for a younger child.

44. (3) This is the protest (first) stage of separation anxeity. Because this is an expected reaction to hospitalization at this age, it may also be considered normal, but this is not as specific an answer as (3).

45. (3) Small amounts of liquid are tolerated better, preventing gastric distention and impingement on the diaphragm causing further distress. Large amounts of fluids are lost through the respiratory tract with increased rate and effort, so fluid must be replaced; solids are often not tolerated. Tepid sponge baths are helpful; cold baths are not appropriate.

PSYCHIATRIC NURSING

1. A depressed client refuses to get out of bed, go to activities, or participate in any of the unit's programs. The most appropriate nursing action is to

   1 Tell her the rules of the unit are that no client can remain in bed.
   2 Suggest she better get out of bed or she will go hungry later.
   3 Tell her that the nurse will assist her out of bed and help her to dress.
   4 Allow her to remain in bed until she feels ready to join the other clients.

2. A young adult is admitted to the hospital for a diagnostic work up. She has recently lost weight and has not had a menstrual period for 3 months. While collecting data, the nurse will focus on a(n)

   1 Interpersonal relationship.
   2 Eating disorder.
   3 Hormone irregularity.
   4 Diet consultation.

3. When encouraged to join an activity, a depressed client on the psychiatric unit refuses and says, "What's the use?" The approach by the nurse that would be most effective is to

   1 Sit down beside her and ask her how she is feeling.
   2 Tell her it is time for the activity, help her out of the chair, and go with her to the activity.
   3 Convince her how helpful it will be to engage in the activity.
   4 Tell her that this is a self-defeating attitude and it will only make her feel worse.

4. When a depressed client becomes more active and there is evidence that her mood has lifted, an appropriate goal to add to the nursing care plan is to

   1 Encourage her to go home for the weekend.
   2 Move her to a room with three other clients.
   3 Monitor her whereabouts at all times.
   4 Begin to explore the reasons she became depressed.

5. A client with a history of alcohol abuse is admitted to the emergency room with delirium tremens (DTs). The physician orders Valium 10 mg, IV with vitamin B_6, vital signs every 30 minutes, regular diet, environment with no stimuli. Which intervention will the nurse implement first?

   1 Vital signs.
   2 Valium 10 mg.
   3 IV with vitamin B_6.
   4 Quiet environment.

6. When a client's hallucinations become more insistent, demanding, and difficult to ignore, the nurse assesses his mental status as

   1 Improving.
   2 Deteriorating.
   3 Remaining the same.
   4 Showing more evidence of paranoia.

7. During the last 15 years, suicide has increased dramatically in the age group of

   1 Menopausal women.
   2 Adolescents.
   3 Elderly men.
   4 Children under age 12.

8. Group therapy has been an accepted method of treatment for psychiatric clients for several years. The best rationale for this form of treatment is

   1 It is the most economical—one staff member can treat many clients.
   2 The format of the therapy is realistic and does not deal with unconscious material.
   3 It enables clients to become aware that others have problems and that they are not alone in their suffering.
   4 It provides a social milieu similar to society in general, where the client can relate to others and validate perceptions in a realistic setting.

9. A 60-year-old male client has been admitted to the psychiatric unit, with symptoms ranging from fatigue, an inability to concentrate and an inability to complete everyday tasks, to refusal to care for himself and preferring to sleep all day. One of the first interventions should be aimed at

   1 Developing a good nursing care plan.
   2 Talking to his wife for cues to help him.
   3 Encouraging him to join activities on the unit.
   4 Developing a structured routine for him to follow.

10. A client becomes very dejected and states that life isn't worth living and no one really cares what happens to him. The best response from the nurse would be

    1 "Of course, people care. Your wife comes to visit every day."
    2 "Let's not talk about sad things. Why don't we play Ping-pong?"
    3 "I care about you, and I am concerned that you feel so down."
    4 "Tell me, who doesn't care about you?"

11. A female client on a psychiatric unit has just told the nurse that she is thinking of committing suicide. The appropriate intervention would be to

    1 Notify the charge nurse.
    2 Ask the client if she has a plan.
    3 Request special one-to-one observation.
    4 Administer the PRN ordered medication.

12. A nurse observes a client sitting alone in her room crying. As the nurse approaches her, the client states, "I'm feeling sad. I don't want to talk now." The nurse's best response would be

    1 "It will help you feel better if you talk about it."
    2 "I'll come back when you feel like talking."
    3 "I'll stay with you a few minutes."
    4 "Sometimes it helps to talk."

13. A client with the diagnosis of manic episode is racing around the psychiatric unit trying to organize games with the clients. An appropriate nursing intervention is to

    1 Have the client play Ping-Pong.
    2 Suggest video exercises with the other clients.
    3 Take the client outside for a walk.
    4 Do nothing, as organizing a game is considered therapeutic.

14. When assessing a client for possible suicide, an important clue would be if the client

    1 Is hostile and sarcastic to the staff.
    2 Identifies with problems expressed by other clients.
    3 Seems satisfied and detached.
    4 Begins to talk about leaving the hospital.

15. A male client on the psychiatric unit becomes upset when a visitor does not show up, and in a rage, breaks a chair. The first nursing intervention should be to

    1 Stay with the client during the stressful time.

2   Ask direct questions about the client's behavior.

3   Set limits and restrict the client's behavior.

4   Plan with the client for how he can better handle frustration.

16. A client with a diagnosis of obsessive-compulsive disorder constantly does repetitive cleaning. The nurse knows that this behavior is probably most basically an attempt to

1   Decrease the anxiety to a tolerable level.

2   Focus attention on nonthreatening tasks.

3   Control others.

4   Decrease the time available for interaction with people.

17. A client has been admitted with a diagnosis of delirium tremens (DTs). The nurse knows that the primary reason the client is so fearful and apprehensive is because

1   He has a serious mental illness.

2   He may die, as 15 percent of the people with DTs do die.

3   His illusions and hallucinations are very real to him.

4   He has to give up alcohol until the symptoms recede.

18. A client is experiencing a high degree of anxiety. It is important to recognize if additional help is required because

1   If the client is out of control, another person will help to decrease his anxiety level.

2   Being alone with an anxious client is dangerous.

3   It will take another person to direct the client into activities to relieve anxiety.

4   Hospital protocol for handling anxious clients requires at least two people.

19. A 56-year-old client is tentatively diagnosed as having Korsakoff's syndrome. In developing a strategy to care for this client, the nurse knows that this condition is a/an

1   Neurological condition common with alcohol poisoning.

2   Neurological degeneration caused by vitamin deficiency.

3   Organic brain lesion brought on by repeated hepatitis attacks.

4   State resulting from severe, long-term psychosis.

20. Three days after admission for depression, a 54-year-old female client approaches the nurse and says, "I know I have cancer of the uterus. Can't you let me stay in bed and have some peace before I die?" In responding, the nurse must keep in mind that

1   The client must be postmenopausal.

2   Thoughts of disease are common in depressed clients.

3   Clients suffering from depression can be demanding, making many requests of the nurse.

4   Antidepressant medications frequently cause vaginal spotting.

21. As a depressed client begins to participate in her treatment program, an indication that she is ready for discharge will be when she has

1   Formulated a plan to return home and continue therapy.

2   Talked to her boss about returning to work.

3   Identified her weak areas and is working on them.

4   Asked the staff for advice about her future.

22. A client with Alzheimer's disease is talking to the tree in the corner of the room as if it were a person. An appropriate intervention would be to

1   Tell the client that he is talking to a tree.

2   Ignore the incident.

3   Write the incident in the chart.

4   Begin a conversation with the client.

23. The nurse observes a client's daughter, who is visiting her mother, sitting alone and crying. When approached, the daughter states, "I'm really concerned about Mom." The nurse's best response would be

1 "Are you concerned about her hospitalization?"
2 "Tell me what's concerning you."
3 "Would you like to talk with the social worker?"
4 "Would you like to talk to her physician?"

24. Of the following approaches to a client with organic brain syndrome, the most therapeutic would be to

1 Use short, concrete, specific interactions.
2 Give complete explanations to the client about his problems.
3 Provide a flexible therapy schedule.
4 Confront the client whenever he loses contact with reality.

25. In assisting in the treatment of a person on a "bad trip" from LSD ingestion, the nurse would

1 Stay with the client.
2 Ask him what help he would like to have.
3 Encourage verbalization of feelings and perceptions.
4 Provide ongoing orientation.

26. A schizophrenic client is admitted to the psychiatric unit. As the nurse approaches the client with medication, he refuses it, accusing the nurse of trying to kill him. The nurse's best strategy would be to tell him that

1 "It is not poison and you must take the medication."
2 "I will give you an injection if necessary."
3 "You may decide if you want to take the medication by mouth or injection, but you must take it."
4 "It's all right if you don't take the medication right now."

27. An elderly, depressed client has orders for electroconvulsive therapy (ECT). Of the medications administered, the primary purpose of a muscle relaxant is to

1 Decrease anxiety before ECT.
2 Reduce complications from the procedure.
3 Reduce tension in the client's muscles.
4 Block vagal stimulation.

28. A client with the diagnosis of organic brain syndrome, dementia type, confabulates when talking with the nurse. The nurse's best response and the rationale for it is to

1 Tell him she knows he is distorting the situation and not telling the truth because she knows alcoholics need to have moral values reinforced.
2 Sit him down and repeatedly give him the correct version of his activity until he remembers it, because one way of learning is to have something repeatedly stressed.
3 Constantly reiterate the correct story each time he confabulates because a realistic goal with this client is to correct memory distortion.
4 Accept his stories without challenge as he is unable, because of organic damage, to recall accurately.

29. A 50-year-old client has just been admitted to the psychiatric unit with a diagnosis of depression. The nurse can best approach her by saying

1 "You have just been admitted, and I'd like to show you the unit."
2 "Would you like to come with me to occupational therapy and see if you can find a project you would enjoy?"
3 "My name is Mary. I will introduce you to all of the other clients."
4 "My name is Mary. I am a nurse on this floor and I will be spending some time with you."

30. A client has been in the hospital for 3 weeks. His diagnosis is paranoid ideation. The nurse will know that the client's condition is improving when he

    1 Stops talking about the paranoid ideas.
    2 Says that he wants to go home.
    3 Asks the nurse if his ideas are real.
    4 Describes his paranoid ideas to the nurse in great detail.

31. An antisocial client refuses to participate in unit activities, staying in his room reading until late at night. When he is on the unit, he makes fun of the other clients, calling them "nuts" or "stupid." Considering his diagnosis and behavior, the nursing plan that would be most effective for the staff to follow is to

    1 Let the client know the rules on the unit.
    2 Allow the client to isolate himself so that he does not upset the other clients.
    3 Confer with the client, the staff, and his psychiatrist about his lack of participation on the unit.
    4 Require the client's participation in activities.

32. A client with a diagnosis of schizophrenia who threatened a neighbor with a knife was placed on a 72-hour hold by the courts and the psychiatrist. The hold is up, and the psychiatrist and court must determine if the client is

    1 Gravely disabled and unable to take care of himself.
    2 A danger to himself and others.
    3 Able to pay for his hospitalization and treatment.
    4 Willing to remain in treatment if he is discharged.

33. A client tells the nurse that she is having a great deal of difficulty talking to her husband. She says, "He treats me like a child. Nothing I say seems to matter to him." The best response is

    1 "Tell me more about how you and your husband communicate."
    2 "How do you feel about his reactions to you?"
    3 "He sounds very childish himself."
    4 "Why do you think he treats you like a child?"

34. As a male nurse is coming on duty, one of the clients meets him in the elevator and says, "You look like a wreck today." The best response would be

    1 "You don't look so good yourself."
    2 "If you can't say anything nice, perhaps you shouldn't say anything at all."
    3 "I don't understand what you mean by that."
    4 "I was a little rushed this morning."

35. The nurse is in the day room with a group of clients when a client who has been quietly watching TV suddenly jumps up screaming and runs out of the room. The nurse's priority intervention would be to

    1 Turn off the TV, and ask the group what they think about the client's behavior.
    2 Follow after the client to see what has happened.
    3 Ignore the incident because these outbursts are frequent.
    4 Send another client out of the room to check on the agitated client.

36. A client's deafness has been diagnosed as conversion disorder. Nursing interventions should be guided by which one of the following?

    1 The client will probably express much anxiety about her deafness and require much reassurance.
    2 The client will have little or no awareness of the psychogenic cause of her deafness.
    3 The client's need for the symptom should be respected; thus, secondary gains should be allowed.
    4 The defense mechanisms of suppression and rationalization are involved in creating the symptom.

37. A nursing student failed her psychology final exam and spent the entire evening berating the teacher and the course. This behavior would be an example of

    1 Reaction-formation.
    2 Compensation.
    3 Projection.
    4 Acting out.

38. In planning nursing care for the individual with a somatoform or psychosomatic illness, the nurse needs to consider which of the following general concepts?

    1 The nurse must incorporate concepts of adaptation, stress, body image, and anxiety.
    2 The area of symptom formation may be symbolic to the client.
    3 Psychosomatic illnesses may be life threatening.
    4 All of the above concepts are important.

39. The most effective nursing intervention for a severely anxious client who is pacing vigorously would be to

    1 Instruct her to sit down and quit pacing.
    2 Place her in bed to reduce stimuli and allow rest.
    3 Allow her to walk until she becomes physically tired.
    4 Give her PRN medication and walk with her at a gradually slowing pace.

40. A client has been in the hospital for 4 weeks. He is dying of terminal cancer. During this time he has never mentioned his condition or the fact that he is dying. The nurse's knowledge of the dying process leads to the conclusion that the client is

    1 In the grieving process and does not wish to talk.
    2 Still in the denial phase.
    3 Depending on his family for support and talks to them.
    4 Afraid that by talking about dying it will become reality.

41. A new staff nurse is on an orientation tour with the head nurse. A client approaches her and says, "I don't belong here. Please try to get me out." The staff nurse's best response would be

    1 "What would you do if you were out of the hospital?"
    2 "I am a new staff member, and I'm on a tour. I'll come back and talk with you later."
    3 "I think you should talk with the head nurse about that."
    4 "I can't do anything about that."

42. A client on the psychiatric unit frequently gets out of control and is inappropriately aggressive. A plan to teach this client how to cope would include

    1 A problem-solving focus involving alternative responses.
    2 Confronting the client about this behavior.
    3 Informing the client of the consequences of his behavior (i.e., restraints).
    4 Frequent times in seclusion as a part of a behavior modification program.

43. A client is admitted with the diagnosis of alcoholism. The initial goal of the treatment program would be to

    1 Set limits on the client's behavior.
    2 Re-establish a healthy physical condition.
    3 Determine what circumstances led to the condition.
    4 Use group psychotherapy as the primary method of treatment.

44. A client in the hospital asks the nurse what the drug Prozac is used for. The best response would be

    1 "You had better ask your physician."
    2 "It is given for depression. Why do you ask?"
    3 "It is an antidepressant medication that has fewer side effects than other drugs."
    4 "Why are you asking about Prozac?"

45. A client is admitted to the hospital with the diagnosis of narcotic addiction–heroin. In collecting data on the client, the nurse knows
that the effect of this drug on the client is

1   Sedative.
2   Stimulating.
3   Hallucinogenic.
4   A sense of well-being.

PSYCHIATRIC NURSING

Answers with Rationale

1. (3) Be positive, definite and specific about expectations. Do not give depressed clients a choice or try to convince them to get out of bed. Physically assist the client to get up and dressed to mobilize her.

2. (2) Weight loss and no menstrual period for 3 months are symptoms of anorexia nervosa, so an eating disorder should be assessed. This could be the cause of hormone irregularity. Diet consultation would be part of the treatment plan.

3. (2) The nursing intervention is directed toward mobilizing the client without asking her to make a decision or trying to convince her to go. The nurse must be direct, specific and not take no for an answer.

4. (3) The goal is to implement suicide precautions because the danger of suicide is when the depression lifts and the client has the energy to formulate a plan. The nurse would not encourage her to go home where she could not be observed constantly. She could be moved into a room with other clients, but this is not the priority concern.

5. (3) The most important order to implement first is fluids (IV) with B_6 supplement. The main cause of an alcoholic going into DTs is lack of nutrients, especially vitamin B_6. This client also requires the glucose supplement from the IV fluids. The other orders would then be implemented.

6. (2) The more demanding and absorbing hallucinations (hearing voices) become, the more the client's condition may be deteriorating. Secondarily, this may indicate increased paranoia. Paranoid schizophrenia is only one form of this condition, and hallucinations occur in all types of schizophrenia.

7. (2) The number of suicides has increased dramatically in the adolescent age group in the last 15 years. As more elderly are living longer, the number of suicides has also increased, but it is proportional.

8. (4) Because many people's problems occur in an interpersonal framework, the group setting is a way to correct faulty perceptions, as well as to work on more effective ways of relating to others.

9. (4) While a good nursing care plan is important, the priority would be to get the client mobilized. Even without a specific diagnosis, the nurse will realize that part of what is happening with the client is a depressed mood. Providing a structured plan of activities for the client to follow will help his mood to lift and provide a focus so that he will not be centered on internal suffering.

10. (3) A depressed person needs to experience that someone is concerned for his welfare and that there is a person he can relate to during his hospitalization. Answers (1) and (2) negate the client's feelings and answer (4) may focus

on uncomfortable thoughts that will deepen the depression.

11. (2) The most appropriate intervention is to follow through with the client and ask if she has a plan. The client may tell the nurse her plan which would assist in formulating the treatment options. After this, the nurse would notify the charge nurse and request suicide observation.

12. (3) Simply offering comfort by staying with the client and being open for communication is the most therapeutic. The other responses place an additional burden on the client if she does not wish to talk.

13. (3) Engaging the client in a large muscle activity, like walking with the nurse, will direct the client's energy but not be too stimulating, as would a competitive game such as Ping-Pong.

14. (3) Most suggestible of suicide is the sudden sense of satisfaction or relief (perhaps from finally making the decision to commit suicide) and detachment. Hostility, identifying with others, or thinking of the future do not as clearly suggest suicidal thinking.

15. (3) The first intervention is to set firm, clear limits on his behavior. The nurse would also remain with the client until he calms down and then encourage him to discuss his feelings rather than act out.

16. (1) The primary reason for the compulsive activity is to decrease the anxiety caused by obsessive thoughts. The client is not trying to focus her attention on tasks, control others or lessen interaction with others.

17. (3) A client experiencing DTs may have illusions and/or hallucinations. These are very frightening to him because they seem real and the client does not recognize that they are part of his illness.

18. (1) If the client and/or the situation gets out of control, anxiety will only increase. Additional help may prevent this from occurring.

19. (2) Korsakoff's syndrome (also called polyneuritic psychosis) is a form of organic brain syndrome that is associated with long term alcohol abuse and a deficiency of vitamin B complex, especially thiamine. (2) is more specific than answer (1). This condition is not caused from a lesion, hepatitis (3), or psychosis (4).

20. (2) Concern with having a life-threatening disease is a common issue with depressed clients. While demanding behavior may be a symptom, it is not the issue here. Whether or not the client is postmenopausal is not relevant.

21. (1) A plan to return home and continue therapy shows that the client has begun to realistically and responsibly deal with her problems. Talking to her boss is positive but not as comprehensive as (1). Identifying and working on weak areas usually are intermediate steps toward discharge. In asking the staff for advice, the client is not ready or willing to accept responsibility for herself.

22. (4) The goal is to keep the client in reality as much as possible, so beginning a real conversation is the best intervention. The nurse would also write the incident on the client's chart because it is an indication of his condition.

23. (2) The nurse should offer on-the-spot support to visiting family members. They are important components of the therapeutic process and need assistance in dealing with their thoughts and feelings about the client.

24. (1) Organic brain syndrome clients need specific, concrete instructions and a safe, consistent environment with reality orientation. Confrontation and environmental instability further confuse the client by increasing his anxiety level. Giving too much information is confusing.

25. (1) The client needs to have external stimuli decreased but does not need to be isolated. It is much less traumatic if the nurse remains with the client. Encouraging verbalization or answering questions during this period would not be therapeutic.

26. (3) Giving the client a choice of how he would like to take his medication, while being firm that he must take it, gives the client a sense of control and helps to reduce the power struggle. Telling the client that the medication is not poison will do little to persuade him to comply. Answer (2) would represent a punishment. The client must take his medication; therefore, distractor (4) is not appropriate.

27. (2) The purpose of a muscle relaxant is to reduce complications from convulsions that occur with ECT. This medication would reduce muscle tension, but this answer is not as specific. Atropine is given to block vagal stimulation.

28. (4) Confabulation is filling in memory gaps caused by organic deterioration of brain cells. Attempts to correct stories, re-educate or refute may increase anxiety, thus being unproductive and/or detrimental. It would also lower the client's self-esteem.

29. (4) Acknowledge the client by introducing yourself and start a one-to-one relationship by spending time with her. Let the client know that the nurse cares about her by staying with her.

30. (3) When the client is able to question his ideas or ask if they are real, it is a sign of improvement. Wanting to go home or stopping talking about the paranoid ideas is not necessarily an indication of improvement.

31. (3) In dealing with manipulative behavior, it is important that all members of the team and the client are clear about expectations. (1) is nontherapeutic as it pits the nurse against the client. (2) is not a reasonable choice because the client is not involved in treatment. (4) is nontherapeutic.

32. (2) The staff and court must determine if the client is a danger to self and others. Answer (1) may be a correct answer, but the client was admitted to the hospital for threatening a neighbor. Answers (3) and (4) are not pertinent to the decision.

33. (2) The client needs to recognize her feelings, and this response will assist her to do so. Answer (1) keeps the conversation on the cognitive level and does not deal with her feelings. (3) is making a judgment. (4) is asking for an intellectual analysis which may or may not help the client and which may cause her to feel she must justify herself.

34. (3) Asking for clarification of such a statement might reveal more feelings than implied

by the casual comment. This type of statement may be indicative of anger or projected feelings. Answer (1) is sarcastic, and (2) and (4) cut off further exploration of what the client may really be saying. It would not be appropriate to continue with a personal explanation of why the nurse looks bad.

35.   (2)   The immediate priority is to find the client and assess what further intervention may be needed. Whether or not the behavior has happened frequently in the past is irrelevant, because the behavior exhibited now is significant and should be followed up. Sending another client is inappropriate as an immediate intervention may be necessary.

36.   (2)   This disorder has an unconscious mechanism in place; thus, there is a relative lack of distress or anxiety regarding the symptom. The client is likely to demonstrate "la belle indifference," an unconcerned, indifferent attitude toward the loss of function with no awareness of the psychogenic cause. Answer (3) is incorrect as secondary gains should be minimized. Answer (4) is incorrect as repression and displacement are the operating mechanisms.

37.   (3)   The client is placing blame on others and not taking responsibility for her own behavior. Reaction-formation is preventing "dangerous" feelings from being expressed by exaggerating the opposite attitude. Compensation is covering up a weakness by emphasizing a desirable trait. Acting out is not a defense mechanism.

38.   (4)   Psychosomatic illnesses involve the "holism" of the individual; thus, all three of the concepts are important. If the nurse considers all of these concepts in planning nursing care, interventions will be therapeutic.

39.   (4)   This client is in severe anxiety heading for a panic level. She requires immediate medication, constant attention, and a gradual lessening of activity according to her expressed level of energy. With moderate anxiety, directed activity helps to reduce the level.

40.   (2)   The fact that he has not talked about dying in a month, or even about his illness, leads the nurse to suspect denial. In this situation, the nurse would not confront him with reality but wait until he is ready to talk.

41.   (2)   As a new staff member, the nurse should clarify who she is and why she is there. She also should acknowledge the client's attempt to initiate interaction by offering to talk at a more appropriate time. Answer (1) might be used in a later interaction, but is not appropriate at this time.

42.   (1)   The most effective method is problem-solving, allowing the client to explore his feelings, responses, consequences, and try out new, alternative responses. Confrontation may only increase the maladaptive behavior. Threatening the client with restraints or putting him in seclusion is punitive, not creating a climate where he would learn new behavior.

43.   (2)   The first step in the treatment plan would be to focus on the physical condition of the client—to provide a healthy diet with vitamin supplements (these clients are usually low in vitamin B); and adequate rest and sleep. Setting limits, providing structure, and group psychotherapy would be implemented later.

44.   (2)   It is therapeutic to answer the question, then make an open-ended response to en-

courage the client to talk. Answers (1) and (3) close off communication, and (4) does not answer the question.

45. (1) Narcotics like heroin or morphine have a sedative effect on the central nervous system. Cocaine is a stimulant and LSD is hallucinogenic. Marijuana gives one a sense of well-being.

PHARMACOLOGY

1. A client is receiving lithium carbonate for manic behavior. Administration of this medication should be guided by

   1 Maintaining a therapeutic dose of 900 mg TID.
   2 Encouraging regular blood studies (serum lithium levels) until the maintenance dose is stabilized.
   3 Telling the client that a lag of 7 to 10 days can be expected between the initiation of lithium therapy and the control of manic symptoms.
   4 Telling the client that muscle weakness indicates severe toxicity and the physician should be notified.

2. Which of the following actions is *not* accurate when administering a medication using the Z-track method?

   1 Placing 0.3 to 0.5 mL of air into the syringe.
   2 Using a 2- to 3-inch needle.
   3 Inserting the needle and injecting medication without aspirating.
   4 Pulling skin laterally away from the injection site before inserting the needle.

3. The nurse is counseling a client taking corticosteroids who has developed an infectious process. How would the infection affect the medication dosage?

   1 Corticosteroid dose would be increased.
   2 Corticosteroid dose would be discontinued.
   3 Corticosteroid dose would be decreased.
   4 There would be no change in dosage.

4. The nurse is assigned to a client who is receiving mydriatic eye drops. Of the following symptoms, which indicates a systemic anticholinergic effect?

   1 Complaints of light headedness and headache.
   2 Respirations becoming more shallow.
   3 Sweating and blurred vision.
   4 Decreased pulse and blood pressure.

5. A client with a fractured right hip has Buck's traction applied and orders for prophylactic anticoagulant therapy. The nurse anticipates that the physician will order

   1 Aspirin.
   2 Dextran.
   3 Heparin.
   4 Coumadin.

6. When administering a one-time dose of Valium (a benzodiazepine drug) to a client, the nurse needs to consider that

   1 Valium has sedative properties.
   2 There are no important side effects to consider because it is a one-time dose.
   3 Valium should never be mixed with foods containing tyramine.
   4 Valium directly affects the blood pressure as a vasoconstrictor.

7. A female client with a history of multiple sclerosis has orders for dantrolene sodium (Dantrium). The nurse will know the client understands the action of the drug when she says

   1 "I need to use a sunscreen when I go outside."
   2 "I can't take any other medications when I'm on this drug."
   3 "I take this drug only when my spasms are bad."
   4 "I should see a marked change in my muscle strength within 2 to 3 days."

8. A client with a urinary tract infection is given aminoglycoside (Gentamicin) antimicrobial therapy. The nurse understands that this drug is more active when the urine is

1 Concentrated.
2 Dilute.
3 Alkaline.
4 Acid.

9. The instructions to a client whose physician recently ordered nitroglycerin are that this medication should be taken

1 Every 2 to 3 hours during the day.
2 Before every meal and at bedtime.
3 At the first indication of chest pain.
4 Only when chest pain is not relieved by rest.

10. Which one of the statements is most accurate about the drug cimetidine (Tagamet) and should be discussed with clients who take the medication?

1 Tagamet should be taken with an antacid to decrease GI distress, a common occurrence with the drug.
2 Tagamet should be used cautiously with clients on Coumadin because it could inhibit the absorption of the drug.
3 Tagamet should be taken on an empty stomach for better absorption.
4 Tagamet is usually prescribed for long-term prevention of gastric ulcers.

11. A 40 year old client admitted for a diagnostic workup has orders for Seconal at bedtime. The nurse's understanding of this drug is that it has the effect on the body of

1 Tranquilization.
2 Sedation.
3 Mood elevation.
4 Stimulation.

12. Some clients with severely active lupus erythematosus are managed with steroids. A pos-

itive response to steroid therapy would be evidenced by

1 An increase in platelet count.
2 A normal gamma globulin count.
3 A decrease in anti-DNA titer.
4 Negative syphilis serology.

13. A client has developed agranulocytosis as a result of medications he is taking. In counseling the client, the nurse knows that one of the most serious consequences of this condition is

1 The potential danger of excessive bleeding even with minor trauma.
2 Generalized ecchymosis on exposed areas of the body.
3 High susceptibility to infection.
4 Extreme prostration.

14. A client in liver failure from cirrhosis with ascites is receiving spironolactone. The expected outcome when this drug is given is

1 Increased urine sodium.
2 Increased urinary output.
3 Decreased potassium excretion.
4 Prevention of metabolic alkalosis.

15. After a client begins taking a prescribed antianxiety agent, the nurse would observe her for side effects of

1 Sedation and slurred speech.
2 Photosensitivity and muscular rigidity.
3 Tremors and hypertension.
4 A paradoxical reaction and hypoactivity.

16. A client is to receive meperidine (Demerol) 75 mg and atropine 0.2 mg IM. The medications can be mixed together in the same syringe. On hand is Demerol 50 mg per 1 mL and atropine 0.3 mg per 1 mL. What should be the total volume of the two drugs when mixed together into a syringe?

1 1.3 mL.
2 1.6 mL.

3   2.2 mL.

4   2.7 mL.

17.   The client's physician orders 20 mEq of KCl. The label on the KCl is 10 mEq/5 mL. The nurse will give the client

1   10 mL.

2   2 mL.

3   5 mL.

4   20 mL.

18.   A male client is currently taking Digitalis 0.25 mg daily, Lasix 100 mg daily, Acyclovir 10 mg QID, and Tagamet 300 mg QID. Which one of the following drugs has potential side effects that are the most life-threatening?

1   Digitalis.

2   Lasix.

3   Acyclovir.

4   Tagamet.

19.   A 60-year-old male client with chronic osteoarthritis is severely debilitated. Betamethasone (Celestone) therapy has been ordered for him. The nurse will advise the client to take a single, daily dose of the drug

1   At bedtime with a glass of milk.

2   With orange juice at bedtime.

3   With milk in the morning.

4   On an empty stomach in the morning.

20.   A 68-year-old client has an IV infusing at 50 mL per hour. The IV administration set delivers 15 gtts/mL. When adjusting the flow rate, the nurse would regulate the rate at

1   4 drops per minute.

2   8 drops per minute.

3   12 drops per minute.

4   25 drops per minute.

PHARMACOLOGY

Answers with Rationale

1. (3) There will be 7 to 10 days before the client will experience a decrease in the manic symptoms. A therapeutic dose is 300 mg TID; regular blood studies must be continued throughout drug therapy; muscle weakness is an expected side effect and does not indicate toxicity.

2. (3) Pulling back on the plunger, or aspirating, would ensure that the needle had not entered a blood vessel. Therefore, this action would be included in the Z-track method.

3. (1) Infectious processes increase the body's need for steroids. During times of stress (infection) the dose needs to be increased to prevent adrenal insufficiency in previously steroid-dependent clients.

4. (3) Sweating and blurred vision are signs of a systemic anticholinergic effect. In addition to these symptoms the client may experience loss of sight, difficulty breathing, flushing, or eye pain. If these symptoms occur, the medication must be discontinued and the physician notified.

5. (3) Anticoagulant prophylaxis would be initiated with intermittent heparin therapy which is effective immediately. Dextran is frequently given postoperatively and aspirin is used in the recovery period during hospitalization to prevent venous thrombosis.

6. (1) Valium has sedative properties, and the client needs to be warned about possible side effects. For example, driving while taking Valium is dangerous. It is also important to inform the client about the life-threatening danger of mixing this drug with alcohol.

7. (1) This drug has the potential for photosensitivity; therefore, the client should protect her skin by wearing a hat and using sunscreen.

8. (3) Aminoglycoside antibiotics are more active when the urine is alkaline and the client may receive soda bicarbonate to accomplish creating this environment.

9. (3) Nitroglycerin should be taken whenever the client feels a full, pressure feeling or tightness in his chest, not waiting until chest pain is severe. It can also be taken prophylactically before engaging in an activity known to cause angina in order to prevent an anginal attack.

10. (2) Tagamet can interfere with the absorption of Coumadin and several other drugs such as Dilantin, Lidocaine or Inderal; therefore, the serum levels of the drugs should be monitored closely. Tagamet should not be taken within 1 hour of an antacid, because this will interfere with the absorption. It is best to take the drug with food. Tagamet is usually ordered for short-term treatment of duodenal and active gastric ulcers.

11. (2) Seconal is a common barbiturate used for sleeplessness. It has a sedative effect on the CNS. Its use should be monitored be-

cause of potential addiction or overdose, especially with the elderly.

12. (3) Anti-DNA antibody levels correlate most specifically with lupus disease activity. A positive response to steroids would show a decrease in these levels. Twenty percent of clients with lupus develop a positive syphilis serology, and many have hypergammaglobulinemia and a decreased platelet count.

13. (3) Agranulocytosis is characterized by neutropenia (decreased number of lymphocytes) which lowers the body defenses against infection. Granulocytes are the first barrier to infection in the body.

14. (1) The primary action of spironolactone is to increase urine sodium and thereby cause diuresis. It is also potassium sparing and helps counteract metabolic alkalosis by this mechanism.

15. (1) Sedation and slurred speech are the primary side effects. Photosensitivity, an increased susceptibility to sunlight and sunburn, is a common side effect of antipsychotic medications. Muscular rigidity is not a side effect of these medications; in fact, the antianxiety agents often act as muscle relaxants.

16. (3) This computation can be done using the formula D (dose desired) divided by H (dose on hand) multiplied by V (volume). Step I: Compute Demerol dose: 75 divided by 50 multiplied by 1 equals 1.5. Step II: Compute atropine dose: 0.2 divided by 0.3 multiplied by 1 equals 0.66 rounded to 0.7. Step III: Add Demerol and atropine doses: 1.5 plus 0.7 equals 2.2 mL.

17. (1) 10 mL. To calculate the KCl, use the equation: 20 mEq = x mL; because 10 mEq = 5 mL, calculate 10:20:: 5:x; therefore x = 10 mL.

18. (2) Although each of these drugs has significant side effects, Lasix has the potential for life-threatening cardiac arrhythmias. Potassium is lost as a result of the drug use. 100 mg is a large dose and, thus, a low serum potassium level could easily occur leading to ventricular arrhythmias.

19. (3) A single dose in the morning promotes better results and less toxicity. It is given with milk to reduce gastrointestinal irritation.

20. (3) To calculate the drip factor, multiply the hourly rate times the drop factor (50 mL times 15). Divide the answer by 60 minutes (750 / 60 = 12.5 gtts/min). Round off answer to 12.

NUTRITION

1. A client has had abdominal surgery and the physician has ordered a bland diet 3 days post-surgery. Which of the following diet trays would have portions removed because it does not adhere to the dietary regimen?

   1 Scrambled eggs, cereal and white toast.
   2 Baked potato, cottage cheese and coffee.
   3 Cream soup, jello and white toast.
   4 Cooked cereal, boiled egg and milk.

2. A client will have a central vein infusion to maintain nutritional status while his gastrointestinal tract is being bypassed. The nurse would expect that the site of catheter insertion for a protein and glucose concentration of 15% would be in the

   1 Jugular vein.
   2 Right subclavian vein.
   3 Right subclavian artery.
   4 Left arm artery access.

3. A client has injured her eyes with a chemical and must have eye patches in place for several weeks. When her food tray arrives, the most helpful nursing intervention would be to

   1 Feed the client or assign a nursing assistant to feed her.
   2 Explain that her tray is here and put her hands on it.
   3 Tell her to think of a clock and describe which food is where and put the fork in her hand.
   4 Ask her if she would prefer a liquid diet.

4. A 53-year-old client with Crohn's disease is placed on total parenteral nutrition (TPN). The fluid in the present TPN bottle should be infused by 8 AM. At 7 AM the nurse observes that it is empty and another TPN bottle has

   not yet arrived on the unit. The nursing action is to attach a bottle of

   1 D_{25} and water.
   2 D_5 and water.
   3 D_{10} and water.
   4 D_{45} and water.

5. The nurse's discharge teaching for a client with acute pancreatitis will include advising him to take a dietary supplement of

   1 Vitamin K.
   2 Fat soluble vitamins.
   3 Vitamin C.
   4 Vitamin B_{12}.

6. The nurse will know that the client understands presurgical instructions for hemorrhoid surgery if his diet is

   1 Low-roughage.
   2 High-fiber.
   3 High-carbohydrate.
   4 Low-fiber.

7. Discharge planning for a client with a partial colectomy will include which one of the following dietary principles?

   1 High residue, force fluids.
   2 Low residue, no dairy products.
   3 High fiber, no spices.
   4 Regular, no dairy products.

8. The nurse's diet instructions for a client with a colostomy will be

   1 According to his own individual needs and similar to his preoperative diet.
   2 Low in fiber with a large amount of fluids.

3 High in fiber with large amounts of fluids and supplemental vitamin K.

4 Elimination of milk products.

9. Which of the following statements would be correct when counseling a client about the postoperative diet he would receive following a simple surgical procedure?

1 A client undergoing major surgery may have a soft diet the day of surgery.

2 Approximately 2800 calories are required daily for general tissue repair, so this will be his caloric intake.

3 Daily fluid intake should be 1500 mL for an uncomplicated surgical procedure.

4 A mechanical, soft diet should be given the first postoperative day.

10. The nurse will know the client understands his low-purine diet when he states

1 "I will limit the number of fruit servings each day."

2 "Organ meats must be eliminated from my diet."

3 "I can only drink white wine because red wine is high in purine."

4 "Beef, chicken and pork are high in purine; therefore, I can only have them once in a while."

11. The nurse will know that the diabetic client understands his diet when he says that he should obtain the greatest percentage of calories from

1 Fats.

2 Complex carbohydrates.

3 Simple carbohydrates.

4 Protein.

12. The most appropriate sugar substitute for the Insulin-Dependent Diabetes Mellitus, type I (IDDM) client is

1 Corn sugar.

2 Honey.

3 Aspartame.

4 Fructose.

13. A client with acute pancreatitis required nasogastric tube intubation due to persistent vomiting and paralytic ileus. Following NG tube removal, oral feeding should include foods that are

1 High in fat.

2 High in protein.

3 High in carbohydrate.

4 Clear liquid.

14. A client with cirrhosis and ascites is placed on a sodium restricted diet to help control the ascites. In order for this plan to be effective, it is important that the client also

1 Restrict his fluid intake.

2 Increase his potassium intake.

3 Increase his fluid intake.

4 Decrease his potassium intake.

15. A client with a history of pancreatitis should avoid which of the following foods?

1 Noodles.

2 Vegetable soup.

3 Baked fish fillet.

4 Cheddar cheese sandwiches.

16. The nurse questions the dietary department about the lunch delivered for a client with the diagnosis of cirrhosis when she finds on his tray

1 A tuna sandwich.

2 French fries.

3 A ham sandwich.

4 A milkshake.

17. The nurse will know that her teaching has been effective when the client responds that a low fiber diet allows the inclusion of

1 Whole grain breads, seeds and legumes.

2   Fresh fruits and vegetables.

3   Bran and whole grain cereals.

4   Cooked vegetables, fruits and refined breads.

18. Clients with hepatitis may have a regular diet ordered, unless they become increasingly symptomatic. The diet will then be modified to decrease the amount of

    1   Carbohydrates.
    2   Fats.
    3   Fluids.
    4   Protein.

19. A pregnant client client comes to the clinic and the nurse is responsible for nutritional counseling. When the client says that she has eliminated all salt from her diet, the nurse should respond

1   "That's good. Salt is not healthy."

2   "What information did you have that led to this decision?"

3   "At this time we do not advise limiting salt intake."

4   "You can have all the salt you want."

20. Evaluating the teaching plan for a client recently placed on a low sodium diet by her physician, the nurse will know the client understands the plan when she states

    1   "I will call the dietitian if I can't remember."
    2   "I will look at the list of foods I can have."
    3   "I will read the label on the food product."
    4   "I will cook without adding salt to the food."

NUTRITION

Answers with Rationale

1. (2) Coffee is one food eliminated from a bland diet because it is chemically irritating to the stomach. All of the other foods are allowed on a bland diet. Other foods eliminated are raw, spicy, gas-forming, very hot or very cold foods, alcohol, and carbonated drinks.

2. (2) The most common placement site is the right subclavian vein. The jugular vein might be used as an alternative for high concentration IV infusions, but it is more difficult to access. The arm is used for insertion of an arterial line for arterial blood gas samples and monitoring.

3. (3) The most helpful intervention is to assist the client to help herself, allowing her to be as independent as possible. Feeding her or changing the diet to liquid would not be as therapeutic.

4. (3) In order that the client not experience a sudden drop in blood sugar, the solution nearest most TPN solution concentrations is $D_{10}W$. $D_{25}W$ and D_{45} could cause osmotic diuresis or fluid overload.

5. (2) Because the client will be on a low fat diet to decrease pancreatic activity, he will need supplements of the fat soluble vitamins. A well balanced diet should meet the other nutritional needs.

6. (2) A high-fiber diet produces a soft stool without mechanically irritating the hemorrhoidal area. Foods include bran and complex carbohydrates.

7. (2) The low residue diet will put less strain on the colon and eliminating dairy products initially is important because these products cause mucus.

8. (1) Diets are individualized and clients are generally able to eat the same foods they enjoyed preoperatively. Fresh fruits may cause diarrhea in some, but not all, individuals.

9. (2) A daily intake of 2800 calories is required for usual/general tissue repair, whereas 6000 calories may be required for extensive tissue repair. Fluid intake is 2000 to 3000 mL/day for uncomplicated surgery. Diet progresses from nothing by mouth the day of surgery to a general diet within a few days.

10. (2) Organ meats, wine, yeast, scallops, and mussels are all high in purine and must be eliminated from the diet of the client who has gout.

11. (2) The diabetic's diet should be between 50 and 65 percent carbohydrate calories with only 5 percent of these being sucrose. Fat recommendation is less than 30 percent of calories and protein should be 0.8 mg/kg per day.

12. (3) Aspartame is the only calorie-free sweetener listed; the others are nutritive, their average caloric value being 20 Kcal per teaspoon.

When an equal volume of honey and sugar are compared, honey provides about one and one-third times as many Kcal as does table sugar.

13. (3) Foods that are high in carbohydrate are given, because those with high protein or fat content stimulate the pancreas. Alcohol is forbidden.

14. (1) It is important that fluids be restricted as well, because unrestricted fluid intake leads to a progressive decrease in serum sodium from dilution. Electrolyte imbalance with potential neurologic complications could result.

15. (4) Clients with this condition must not consume foods high in fat content because there are inadequate pancreatic enzymes to digest the fat. High fat content also causes pain 2 to 4 hours after ingestion. Suggested diet is high in carbohydrates.

16. (3) Ham is high in sodium and can increase fluid retention leading to edema. Cirrhosis clients are prone to edema as the osmotic pressures change due to a decrease in plasma albumin.

17. (4) Cooked vegetables and fruits as well as refined breads are included in a low-fiber diet. Bran, fresh fruits and whole grains and seeds are included in a high-fiber diet.

18. (4) With liver cell damage, the liver cannot break down and eliminate the protein. Protein needs to be decreased until symptoms dissipate.

19. (3) Research has indicated that pregnant women require a moderate amount of salt because it is essential in maintaining increased body fluids needed for adequate placental and renal flow as well as tissue requirements. Highly salted foods should still be avoided. Answer (2) is wrong because the client's information is wrong and needs to be corrected.

20. (3) The most appropriate response is answer (3). Clients should be instructed to read labels before purchasing canned, frozen or processed foods because they are usually very high in sodium. A list of foods will provide guidance, but she should know the sodium content of food. Not adding salt to foods when cooking is also important, but not as critical as (3).

ONCOLOGY NURSING

1. A client has just received a report from her physician that describes a tumor that was recently biopsied. If the result she receives is listed as "TO, NO, MO," the client will know that she has

   1 No evidence of a primary tumor, lymph node involvement, and metastasis.
   2 No primary tumor, but evidence of a degree of distant metastasis.
   3 A primary tumor and regional nodes involved.
   4 Carcinoma in situ.

2. The nurse is assessing a client with a radiation implant and observes that the implant has been dislodged. The nurse cannot immediately locate the implant. The first nursing action is to

   1 Search for the implant in the bed covers and place it in a lead container.
   2 Call the charge nurse and bar all visitors from the room.
   3 Pick up the source with a foot-long applicator.
   4 Notify the radiation safety team.

3. A client experiencing severe, intractable pain from cancer complains that the pain medication is not handling the pain at all. The nurse has given the client all of the medicine she can receive. The next nursing action is to

   1 Emotionally support the client and tell her she will receive the next dose of medication as soon as possible.
   2 Contact the charge nurse immediately and intervene on the client's behalf to have the pain dose increased or changed.
   3 Suggest the client try breathing or other alternative techniques to cope with the pain.
   4 Explore the nature of the pain and help the client perceive it in a different way.

4. Cancer is the second major cause of death in this country. What is the first step toward effective cancer control?

   1 Increasing government control of potential carcinogens.
   2 Changing habits and customs that predispose the individual to cancer.
   3 Conducting more mass screening programs.
   4 Educating public and professional people about cancer.

5. In order to educate clients, the nurse should understand that the most common site of cancer for a female is the

   1 Uterine cervix.
   2 Uterine body.
   3 Vagina.
   4 Fallopian tubes.

6. A female client was admitted to the hospital for biopsy of the left breast and a possible mastectomy. The client has just returned from surgery after having a mastectomy with reconstruction on the left side. The nurse will position the client in

   1 Low Fowler's, turned to the affected side.
   2 Semi-Fowler's, affected arm elevated.
   3 Semi-Fowler's, turned to unaffected side.
   4 Prone position.

7. When the nurse is counseling a client about preventive measures for cancer, one of the most important behaviors to emphasize is to

   1 Decrease fat intake.
   2 Avoid exposure to the sun.
   3 Avoid smoking.
   4 Obtain adequate rest and avoid stress.

8. A client has just completed a course in radiation therapy and is experiencing radiodermatitis. The most effective method of treating the skin is to

   1 Wash the area with soap and warm water.
   2 Apply a cream or lotion to the area.
   3 Leave the skin alone until it is clear.
   4 Avoid all creams or lotions to the area.

9. The nurse is teaching a class on cancer prevention and treatment. Of the following symptoms, which one is an early warning sign of cancer?

   1 Heartburn.
   2 Fever, chills and cough.
   3 Change in bowel or bladder habits.
   4 Persistent headache.

10. A 45-year-old client has just been admitted to the hospital for an abdominal hysterectomy following a diagnosis of uterine cancer. Results of lab tests indicate that the client's white blood cell count is 9800/cu mm. The most appropriate intervention is to

    1 Call the operating room and cancel the surgery.
    2 Notify the surgeon immediately.
    3 Take no action as this is a normal value.
    4 Call the lab and have the test repeated.

11. A client has possible malignancy of the colon, and surgery is scheduled. The rationale for administering Neomycin preoperatively is to

    1 Prevent infection postoperatively.
    2 Eliminate the need for preoperative enemas.
    3 Decrease and retard the growth of normal bacteria in the intestines.
    4 Treat cancer of the colon.

12. Of the following screening methods for prevention of cancer, the most important one for the client to be aware of is

    1 Magnetic Resonance Imaging (MRI).
    2 Breast self-examination.
    3 Risk assessment.
    4 Sigmoidoscopy.

13. A female client has a cesium needle implanted in her cervix. She asks the nurse if she may get out of bed to go to the bathroom. The appropriate response is to tell her

    1 She may not get out of bed while the needle is implanted.
    2 She may get out of bed with the nurse's help.
    3 The nurse will have to get a physician's order for her to get out of bed.
    4 She must stay in bed, but she can move around to be more comfortable while the needle is implanted.

14. A client with cancer that has metastasized to the liver is started on chemotherapy. His physician has specified divided doses of the antimetabolite. The client asks why he should take the drug in divided doses. The appropriate response is

    1 "There really is no reason; your doctor just wrote the orders that way."
    2 "This schedule will reduce the side effects of the drug."
    3 "Divided doses produce greater cytotoxic effects on the diseased cells."
    4 "Because these drugs prevent cell division, they are more effective in divided doses."

15. A client is suffering from severe side effects from chemotherapy. She is experiencing nausea, vomiting and anorexia. In addition to antiemetic medications, the nurse might suggest

    1 Eliminating salt and spices in the diet.
    2 Drinking fluids only between, not with, meals.
    3 Low-protein meals.
    4 High-calorie and high-protein supplements.

16. For a client who has received a diagnosis of skin cancer, the type that has the poorest prognosis because it metastasizes so rapidly and extensively via the lymph system is

     1 Basal cell epithelioma.
     2 Squamous cell epithelioma.
     3 Malignant melanoma.
     4 Sebaceous cyst.

17. Alkylating drugs are used as chemotherapeutic agents in cancer therapy. The nurse understands that these drugs stop cancer growth by

     1 Damaging DNA in the cell nucleus.
     2 Interrupting the production of necessary cellular metabolites.
     3 Creating a hormonal imbalance.
     4 Destroying messenger RNA.

18. Antineoplastic drugs are dangerous because they affect normal as well as cancer tissue. Normal cells that divide and proliferate rapidly are more at risk. Which of the following areas of the body would be least at risk?

     1 Bone marrow.
     2 Nervous tissue.
     3 Hair follicles.
     4 Lining of the GI tract.

19. While the nurse is orienting a client scheduled for surgery, the client states she is afraid of what will happen the next day. The most appropriate response is to

     1 Assure her that the surgery is very safe and problems are rare.
     2 Encourage her to talk about her fears as much as she wishes.
     3 Explain that her physician is one of the best and she has nothing to worry about.
     4 Explain that worrying will only prolong her hospitalization.

20. A client has had a partial colectomy. Surgery began at 7:30 AM. She returned to the unit at 1:30 PM. During a 6:00 PM assessment, the nurse observed all of the following. A priority concern that would require the earliest intervention is a

     1 Dressing that is moderately saturated with serosanguineous drainage.
     2 Warm and reddened area on the client's left calf.
     3 Distended bladder that is firm to palpation.
     4 Decrease in breath sounds on the right side.

ONCOLOGY NURSING

Answers with Rationale

1. (1) The staging of the cancer according to cancer classification means that there is no evidence of a primary tumor (TO), regional lymph nodes are not abnormal (NO), and there is no evidence of distant metastasis (MO).

2. (2) The first nursing action is to bar all visitors from the room and notify the charge nurse who will notify the physician. It is important not to contaminate yourself by searching for the implant. The physician will notify the radiation team and make decisions about reimplanting the radiation source in the client.

3. (2) It is the nurse's responsibility to intervene with the charge nurse and physician and report that the pain medication is not providing adequate pain relief. Undertreatment with analgesics has been identified as a major problem for cancer clients, and studies have shown that physicians frequently underprescribe. The other responses will help support the client, but they will not be effective enough to relieve severe pain.

4. (4) The most important step in controlling cancer is educating the public about cancer and its warning signs. Education will have an effect on early diagnosis and treatment.

5. (1) Cervical cancer is the most common site and squamous cell CA is the most common cell type.

6. (2) The most therapeutic position is semi-Fowler's with the affected arm elevated to prevent edema and promote drainage. The client should be turned only to the back and unaffected side.

7. (3) Avoiding smoking is a primary cancer preventive behavior. Smoking is believed to be the cause of 75 percent of lung cancers in the United States. All of the other behaviors are also important preventive measures, but tobacco is a known carcinogen.

8. (4) Irradiated areas are very sensitive; all creams and lotions, which would serve to irritate the skin, should be avoided. The area should be washed with lukewarm water; a mild soap may be used, but most physicians prefer clear water.

9. (3) A change in bowel or bladder habits is one of the seven early warning signs of cancer. Indigestion or difficulty swallowing is a sign, as is a nagging cough or hoarseness.

10. (3) The normal WBC count is 5000 to 10,000 per cu mm. If the results were abnormally high or low, the surgeon would have to be notified and the surgery may be canceled. Tests with abnormal results are not routinely repeated unless the results are grossly abnormal.

11. (3) Neomycin suppresses normal bacterial flora, thereby "sterilizing" the bowel preoperatively to decrease the possibility of postopera-

tive infection. It cannot prevent infection. Neomycin does not influence the need for preoperative enemas or treat cancer of the colon.

12. (2) Breast self-examination (BSE) is the most important method to instruct the client about because it is a primary prevention method. It is performed every month (whereas a mammogram is done every year after age 50), and many breast lumps are first found by the woman when she is examining her breasts. An MRI would be done for diagnosis. Risk assessment and sigmoidoscopy are also important preventive measures, but in priority fall below a BSE.

13. (1) While the sealed source is implanted, the client must remain on bedrest, and movement is restricted to prevent dislodging the radiation source. The client must remain on her back and should not turn or move in bed.

14. (3) Because not all cells will be in the same phase at the same time, divided doses will produce greater cytotoxic effects. This schedule will not reduce the side effects of the drug. Even though the drugs may prevent cell division, divided doses will not affect this characteristic.

15. (4) The most effective deterrent to the nausea and vomiting is to offer the client high-calorie and high-protein supplements. If diarrhea is a problem, eliminating spices would be helpful. Food preferences of the client may also encourage eating (additional seasoning; small, more frequent meals; etc.). Not including fluids with meals may be helpful, but it is not known to help nausea and vomiting.

16. (3) Malignant melanoma has the poorest prognosis. Basal cell epithelioma and squamous cell epithelioma are both superficial, easily excised, slow-growing tumors. A sebaceous cyst is a benign (nonmalignant) growth.

17. (1) Alkylating agents affect production of DNA which, in turn, disrupts cell growth and division.

18. (2) Nervous tissue is least at risk. (1), (3) and (4) are the cells that are most vulnerable because they have rapid cell division and proliferation similar to cancer cells. The nervous tissue cells do not have rapid cell division.

19. (2) Allowing the client to express her fears results in a decrease in anxiety and a more realistic and knowledgeable reaction to the situation. Studies have shown that the less anxiety the client has about the surgery, the more positive the postoperative results. (1) and (3) are false reassurance and nontherapeutic.

20. (3) Inability to void after surgery is a common problem resulting from anesthesia or pain medication and requires an early intervention. It is important to be aware of the client's output for several reasons: to ensure adequate intake, to detect renal problems, and to assess for blood pressure problems. Solution to this problem is catheterization, based on a physician's order. The dressing should be closely observed but is not presently a problem. The area on the calf may be developing thrombophlebitis and should be reported to the physician immediately. The breath sounds can be improved by turning, coughing and deep breathing.

GERONTOLOGY NURSING

1. A client has been admitted to the orthopedic unit with an intracapsular fracture of the right hip sustained after a fall on the ice. Buck's extension is applied and arrangements are being made for hip prosthesis surgery in the morning. The purpose for the application of Buck's extension at this time is to

   1 Reduce the fracture.
   2 Relieve muscle spasms.
   3 Keep the knee extended.
   4 Stabilize the fractured hip.

2. An elderly client with infectious hepatitis (Hepatitis A) and his family are being instructed by the nurse in prevention techniques. The single most important action to prevent this disease is

   1 Not to eat out in public places.
   2 Good personal hygiene.
   3 Thorough handwashing.
   4 Active immunization.

3. The signs of pacemaker malfunction that the nurse would include in discharge teaching for a client with a new pacemaker are

   1 Increased urine output, headache.
   2 Regular, slow pulse.
   3 Weakness, fatigue.
   4 Disorientation, confusion.

4. Serum potassium levels should be evaluated for a client on diuretics. If the potassium level were low, the nurse would expect to find

   1 Dyspnea.
   2 Skeletal muscle weakness.
   3 Hypertension.
   4 Headache.

5. A 70-year-old client with organic brain syndrome, dementia type, is frequently incontinent, even when he is fully dressed. An initial plan to deal with this behavior is to

   1 Remind the client to tell the nurse when he has to urinate.
   2 Put the client in diapers.
   3 Take the client to the bathroom on a 2-hour schedule.
   4 Tell the client that he must remember to go to the bathroom before he wets his pants.

6. After a Foley catheter was inserted for 2 days, it was removed by the nurse. The response considered to be normal at this time is

   1 Dribbling after the first several voidings.
   2 Urgency and frequency for several days.
   3 Frequent voidings in small amounts.
   4 Retention of urine for 10- to 12-hour periods.

7. An elderly female client with newly diagnosed osteoporosis requires counseling prior to discharge. The most important components of the discharge plan are

   1 Instruction in safety factors to prevent injury.
   2 Monitoring medications.
   3 Instruction in regular exercise and diet.
   4 Appropriate use of body mechanics.

8. A 63-year-old male client with a history of alcohol abuse has been admitted with a diagnosis of acute pancreatitis. After completing data collection on the client, the priority nursing diagnosis would be

   1 Fluid volume deficit due to fluid losses into body spaces.

2   Impaired oxygenation due to rapid respirations.

3   Potential for infection due to decreased immune response.

4   Alteration in nutrition, less than requirements, due to decreased intake.

9.   A 78-year-old client who suffered a cerebrovascular accident (CVA) is in a long-term facility. She has developed a pressure ulcer. The nurse is applying a wet-to-damp dressing. The rationale for using this type of dressing is to

1   Prevent the dressing from leaking on the bed clothes.

2   Prevent damage to granulating tissue when removing the dressing.

3   Enable the dressing to almost dry on the ulcer to promote healing.

4   Assist in debriding the wound.

10.   A 60-year-old female client has received the diagnosis of hypertension. Her blood pressure is 160/100. Which of the following symptoms would the nurse expect to find during data collection?

1   Dizziness and flushed face.

2   Drowsiness and confusion.

3   Faintness when getting out of bed.

4   Ataxia and tachycardia.

11.   A client in a long-term care facility has the diagnosis of Alzheimer's disease. His care plan should include the goal of assisting him to participate in activities that provide him a chance to

1   Interact with other clients.

2   Compete with others.

3   Succeed at something.

4   Get a sense of continuity.

12.   A 72-year-old client diagnosed with Meniere's disease has been admitted to the medical-surgical unit. He asks the nurse if he can get up and go to the bathroom any time he needs to. The most appropriate response is

1   "Yes, whenever you wish, you may go."

2   "No, you are on strict bedrest."

3   "Please ring for assistance when you wish to get out of bed."

4   "We will have to check with the physician."

13.   Oxygen is ordered for a 70-year-old client hospitalized for congestive heart failure. Which of the following methods of administration will deliver the highest concentration of oxygen?

1   Venturi mask.

2   Nasal prongs.

3   Oxygen catheter.

4   Mask with reservoir bag.

14.   After the client has recovered from coronary bypass surgery, her physician has advised a low-cholesterol diet. The nurse will know that the client understands this diet when she includes foods such as

1   Meats, especially organ meats, and dairy products.

2   Eggs, cheese, fruits, and vegetables.

3   Vegetables, fruits, lean meats, and vegetable oils.

4   Raw or cooked vegetables, fruits, and red meat.

15.   An elderly client is in a long-term care facility. She had a left-sided CVA 4 weeks ago and has been bedridden since that time. A sign or symptom indicating a possible complication of immobility is

1   A reddened area over the sacrum.

2   Stiffness in the left leg.

3   Difficulty moving her left arm.

4   Difficulty hearing low voices.

16.   A client, age 70, is admitted with the diagnosis of organic brain syndrome, dementia type.

Assessing his condition, the nurse would expect that his prognosis is

1 Good, because the condition tends to be reversible.
2 Unpredictable because the condition may reverse.
3 Poor because symptoms are reduced intellectual capacity, emotional stability, memory, and judgment.
4 Poor because the condition will rapidly progress.

17. An 87-year-old client is admitted to the hospital complaining of weakness and shortness of breath. Her diagnosis is congestive heart failure. As the nurse is assessing the client's condition, which of the following signs will indicate that she is in left-sided heart failure?

1 Fatigue, dyspnea and wheezing.
2 Hepatomegaly and oliguria.
3 Increased pulmonary artery pressure.
4 Peripheral edema such as sacral edema.

18. The visiting home health nurse is assigned to a client who just had cataract surgery. A care plan would include instructions to

1 Maintain bedrest for at least 2 days with bathroom privileges only.
2 Keep the head up and straight and not to look down.
3 Deep breathe and cough four times a day.
4 Only lie on the affected side when in bed.

19. Instructing a 60-year-old client with long-term diabetes on preventing chronic complications of retinopathy or nephropathy, an important principle to teach would be to

1 Visit the physician frequently for check-ups.
2 Obtain frequent lab values of BUN and creatinine.
3 Complete frequent blood glucose testing.
4 Maintain stable blood glucose levels.

20. The nurse is assessing a 75-year-old client who is taking digitalis. The initial clinical symptoms indicating digitalis toxicity would include

1 Anorexia, nausea, vomiting.
2 Diarrhea, headache, vertigo.
3 Nausea, vomiting, diarrhea.
4 Vomiting, diarrhea, vertigo.

GERONTOLOGY NURSING

Answers with Rationale

1. (2) The purpose of Buck's extension application following hip fracture is immobilization to relieve muscle spasm at the fracture site and, thereby, relieve pain. Any movement of fracture fragments will aggravate severe muscle spasm and pain. Skin traction such as this is not used to reduce a fracture and it is not important to keep the knee extended. Bryant's or Russell's traction will stabilize a fractured femur, not the hip.

2. (3) Thorough handwashing is the most important action to prevent the transmission of Hepatitis A. Good personal hygiene is also important, but it does not replace handwashing. Contaminated food is a mode of transmission. Passive immunization is prevention.

3. (3) Weakness and fatigue are symptoms that indicate hypoxia to the tissues. The client should be taught to recognize these as symptoms of pacemaker malfunction.

4. (2) Skeletal muscle weakness is a result of low potassium levels in the blood; potassium is required for normal muscle function. Hypotension may occur, as well as cardiac arrhythmias and tachycardia. Dyspnea and headache are specific indications of hypokalemia.

5. (3) Because the client cannot remember to tell the nurse or remember himself to go to the bathroom, the best plan is to take him on a schedule. This is preferable to dressing him in diapers, even though this may eventually have to be done.

6. (1) Dribbling may be normal until the sphincter muscles regain their tone. If the catheter had been in place for several weeks, (3) might have been the most appropriate response. Urgency and frequency are symptoms of a bladder infection.

7. (3) Because this is a new diagnosis, regular exercise (especially weight-bearing) and a diet high in protein, calcium and vitamin D with avoidance of alcohol and coffee are the most important components of the plan to prevent extension of the condition.

8. (1) Because of the autodigestion of pancreatic and surrounding tissue, there is interstitial hemorrhage, local vascular drainage, increased vascular permeability, and vasodilation. Fluid loss will lead to fluid volume deficit. The client will be placed on bedrest, a nasogastric tube inserted, and analgesics will be used liberally for extreme pain.

9. (2) Wet-to-damp dressings prevent damage to new tissue when dressing is removed. Wet-to-dry dressing debrides the wound (4). This dressing is not to prevent leaking (1) and allowing the dressing to almost dry will not support new tissue.

10. (1) Cardinal symptoms are dizziness and flushed face as well as headache, tinnitus and epistaxis. Drowsiness and confusion occur in hypertensive crisis and faintness would occur in hypotension.

11. (3) It is essential that the client participate in activities that provide him with immediate success and increase his self-esteem. Interaction with others is important but is secondary to improving his self-esteem.

12. (3) The client may be on bedrest (although not strict) due to the extreme vertigo he may experience. Because of the dizziness, he should ring for assistance if he does wish to get up to go to the bathroom. This is a safety intervention to prevent the client from falling.

13. (4) A liter flow of 8 to 10 will provide an FIO_2 of 70 to 100%. The reservoir bag contains a high level of oxygen. As the client inhales, oxygen is taken in from the bag. (1) The Venturi mask delivers a fixed FIO_2, usually 24 to 35%. (2) A 38 to 44% FIO_2 is the maximum amount of oxygen delivered through prongs.

14. (3) These food choices will provide the lowest cholesterol content. Whole milk, dairy products, and fatty meats are all high in cholesterol.

15. (1) A reddened area over the sacrum may be the first sign of a pressure ulcer. If it is recognized at this stage and nursing actions are taken to avoid additional pressure (frequent turning, massaging the skin, etc.), the ulcer may be prevented. Answers (2) and (3) can be expected with left-sided CVA and (4) is usually an expected development with an elderly person.

16. (3) Dementia has a poor prognosis, is usually progressive and irreversible, and the symptoms are closely related to the client's basic personality. All of the characteristics in (3) fit the picture of organic brain syndrome. The condition may or may not progress rapidly, but will generally deteriorate.

17. (1) In left-sided heart failure, congestion occurs mainly in the lungs. It is caused by inadequate ejection of the blood into the systemic circulation. Dyspnea, sneezing, coughing, rales, and fatigue are common symptoms. The other answers refer to right-sided failure.

18. (2) Keeping the head straight and avoiding looking down will prevent increasing intraocular pressure. The nurse would practice breathing exercises with the client but will not encourage coughing, as this could cause an increase in intraocular pressure in the operative eye.

19. (4) The most important principle to teach the client is the necessity of maintaining stable blood glucose levels. Frequent testing is part of the picture but unless the levels are stabilized, testing itself is not enough.

20. (1) Anorexia is the initial symptom associated with digitalis toxicity. Nausea and vomiting are very common symptoms also.

LEGAL ISSUES

1. The requirements for licensure and entry into practice for the practical nurse are determined by the

   1   State Board of Nursing.
   2   American Nurses' Association.
   3   National League for Nursing.
   4   School of Nursing.

2. The nurse's liability in terms of the client's consent to receive health services is to

   1   Be certain that the physician has prepared the client.
   2   Ensure that the client is fully informed before being asked to sign a consent form.
   3   Check that the client understands the details of the surgery.
   4   The nurse would not be liable—the physician would be.

3. Which of the following might negate liability on the part of the nurse in a negligent action?

   1   The client consented to the act.
   2   The harm was not reasonably foreseeable.
   3   The nurse had not been taught to do the procedure in nursing school.
   4   Other foreseeable acts occurred that added to the client's injury.

4. Which of the following statements concerning nursing liability is true?

   1   A physician may assume personal liability for the negligent acts of the nurse.
   2   The nurse is responsible for her own negligent acts.
   3   The doctrine of respondeat superior always protects the nurse.
   4   Malpractice insurance will always cover the damages assessed against the nurse.

5. Client's rights can be defined as

   1   Rights specifically written into many laws.
   2   A position paper that was developed by the American Hospital Association.
   3   A declaration of the World Health Organization.
   4   Rights not supported by statutory law.

6. A state's Nurse Practice Act would *not* include

   1   A definition of nursing practice.
   2   Qualifications for licensure.
   3   Grounds for revocation of a license.
   4   Difference between RN and LVN functions.

7. The nurse is asked to do a TV commercial for hand lotion. In this commercial she will wear her nurse's uniform and advocate the use of this lotion by nurses in their work setting. In doing this the nurse is violating

   1   Consumer fraud laws.
   2   The nurse practice act.
   3   The code of ethics for nurses.
   4   None of the above.

8. For an LVN, which of the following would *not* constitute negligent conduct?

   1   A medication error.
   2   Failure to follow a physician's order.
   3   Failure to challenge a physician's order.
   4   Disagreeing with a physician.

9. The nurse transcribing the physician's order finds it difficult to read. Which of the following people should the nurse consult for clarification of the order?

   1   The head nurse who is familiar with the physician's writing.

2   An RN working with the nurse.

3   The physician who wrote the order.

4   The nursing supervisor.

10.   If the nurse is involved in a situation in which he or she must countersign the charting of a paraprofessional, which of the following will most aid in decreasing legal liability?

1   Read the document before it is signed.

2   Have personal knowledge of the information contained in the document.

3   Make sure the information is accurate.

4   Check with a second nurse to see if information is accurate.

11.   Which of the following best describes the function and purpose of the unusual occurrence (incident) report?

1   A legal part of the chart used to furnish data about the incident.

2   A hospital record used to record the details of the incident for possible legal reference.

3   A legal hospital business record which is subject to subpoena and can be used against the hospital personnel.

4   A hospital record that is entered into the client's chart if he or she dies.

12.   The physician wrote a medication order for a client. The LVN thought the dosage was incorrect. She questioned the physician who said it was all right. Still questioning, she asked the RN, who said it was all right. The LVN gave the medicine, and the client died from an overdose. Who is liable?

1   The physician and the two nurses.

2   The physician.

3   The nurse who gave the medication.

4   Both the physician and the nurse who gave the medication.

13.   The decision as to whether or not a nurse can lawfully restrain a client is made by the

1   Nurse.

2   Family.

3   Hospital administrator.

4   Physician.

14.   One of the elements of negligence is breach of the standard of care. "Standard of care" may be defined as

1   Nursing competence as defined by the State Nurse Practice Act.

2   Degree of judgment and skill in nursing care given by a reasonable and prudent professional nurse under similar circumstances.

3   Health services as prescribed by community ordinances.

4   Giving care to clients in good faith to the best of one's ability.

15.   The primary purpose and criteria of licensure is to

1   Limit practice.

2   Define the scope of practice.

3   Protect the public.

4   Outline legislative action.

16.   The civil rights of a client would not be jeopardized in which one of the following situations?

1   Trying to forcibly detain a client who may suffer great harm by leaving the hospital.

2   Giving emergency medical care to a client without his or her consent or the consent of the family.

3   Giving a psychiatric client's letters addressed to the President of the United Sates to his physician.

4   Giving the client's insurance broker access to his chart.

LEGAL ISSUES

Answers with Rationale

1. (1) Each state creates a board of nursing which defines the scope of practice and establishes the requirements for licensure and entry into practice. Most boards' power is conferred by state statute.

2. (2) The client must be fully informed of potentially harmful effects of the treatment. If this is not done, it could result in the nurse's being personally liable.

3. (2) If basic rules of human conduct are not violated, the elements of liability may not exist. There must be certain elements of liability present; for example, there must exist a causal relationship between harm to the client and the act by the nurse. There must be some damage or harm sustained by the client and there must be a legal basis—such as statutory law—for finding liability.

4. (2) The nurse is responsible for her or his own negligent acts; however, legal doctrine holds that an employer is also liable for negligent acts of employees.

5. (1) All but ten states have some provision for the rights of clients written into a law; and, these rights can be enforced by the law.

6. (4) Each state has their own Nurse Practice Act for RNs and LVNs. Separately, they are a series of statutes enacted by a state to regulate the practice of nursing in that state. It includes all of these plus education.

7. (3) The code of ethics is a set of formal guidelines for governing professional action. This situation is not illegal—it is unethical.

8. (4) Because the nurse is a licensed professional with an education based on a defined body of knowledge, he or she has the right, indeed the responsibility, to disagree with the physician. This is especially so when the health and welfare of the client is involved.

9. (3) Because the nurse will be responsible (and liable) if she transcribes the order incorrectly, the physician who wrote the order should be consulted.

10. (2) To sign a document without having personal knowledge of what occurred would open the possibility of liability.

11. (2) The most accurate answer is (2). The other purposes are to help document the quality of care and to identify areas where more inservice education is needed.

12. (4) The professional nurse, as well as the physician who wrote the order, are held responsible (liable) for harm resulting from their negligent acts.

13. (4) To administer any form of restraint, there must be a physician's order.

14. (2) Nursing actions are evaluated against a set of standards referred to as standards of performance.

15. (3) The primary purpose of licensing nurses, both RN and LVN, is to safeguard the public by determining that the nurse is a safe and competent practitioner.

16. (2) Key elements of a client's rights are consent, confidentiality and involuntary commitment.

VI

COMPREHENSIVE TESTS 3–4

COMPREHENSIVE TEST 3

1. The nurse is assigned a client whose orders include heparin therapy. The substance that the nurse will keep at the bedside as the antidote is

    1 Magnesium sulfate.
    2 Vitamin K.
    3 Protamine sulfate.
    4 Calcium gluconate.

2. The client has arrived in the recovery room following a lobectomy. As the nurse assigned to care for the client during the immediate postoperative period, the first intervention will be to

    1 Take the client's temperature, blood pressure, respirations, and pulse for baseline data.
    2 Check that the IV is running on time and that the correct solution is infusing.
    3 Administer oxygen through an appropriate supply device.
    4 Connect the Pleur-evac to suction.

3. Which nursing behavior is correct when applying a topical transdermal medication patch?

    1 Wipe the planned site of application with alcohol.
    2 Apply the patch to an area that will be covered by clothing.
    3 Gently rub the patch on the skin before taping it down.
    4 Remove the old patch before applying a new one.

4. Important discharge instructions the nurse will give the parents of a child with frequent otitis media would include

    1 Proper administration of antibiotics, pain control, and reporting irritability that deteriorates to lethargy.

    2 Stopping the antibiotics when the acute pain is diminished to prevent developing resistance to the common antibiotics.
    3 Children should be kept away from school and other children until the full course of medication is completed, and their activity restricted.
    4 Avoiding any additional dental work because of the likelihood of recurrence of otitis media.

5. A client has been given the diagnosis of compulsive disorder. As part of her treatment plan, the client will join a daily group therapy session at 10:30 in the morning. The rationale for choosing this time of day is

    1 Anxious clients are more relaxed in the morning.
    2 Mornings are better for group therapy because clients have the rest of the day to work through problems that come up during the sessions.
    3 Most groups are planned for the morning when physicians are on the unit.
    4 The client will have just completed her ritualistic activity.

6. While the IV fluids are infusing via infusion pump, the nurse monitors the system every hour and suspects a significant amount of air has entered the tubing. The first action is to

    1 Immediately shut off the IV and notify the charge nurse.
    2 Increase the drops per minute to flush the air out.
    3 Place the client on his left side.
    4 Place the client in an upright position.

7. After a normal labor and delivery, the infant weighs only 5 pounds and is considered premature. One of the most important principles

in providing nutrition for this premature infant is to

1 Use a regular nipple with a large hole.
2 Feed every 4 to 6 hours.
3 Use a premie nipple for bottle feeding.
4 Use milk high in fat for the formula.

8. The nurse responsible for administering a thiazide medication to a client evaluates his recent lab reports, which are K$^+$ 3.0 and NA$^+$ 140. The nurse would

1 Administer the thiazide drug.
2 Notify the physician.
3 Withhold the drug and have the lab repeat the tests.
4 Withhold the drug and report K$^+$ level to the physician.

9. The best rationale for the nurse introducing her- or himself to a blind client and telling him exactly what care will be administered is to

1 Illustrate the principle of open communication.
2 Decrease the client's anxiety and fear of the unknown.
3 Follow steps for beginning a nurse-client relationship.
4 Encourage and utilize clear communication.

10. The nurse, while admitting a 3-year-old boy to the hospital, observes that he has several garlic cloves hanging from a cord around his neck. What is the appropriate nursing action?

1 Ask the mother to explain the purpose of the garlic.
2 Explain to the mother that the garlic will need to be removed during hospitalization.
3 Teach the mother that it is unsafe for a 3 year old to wear a neck cord.
4 Remove the garlic and assure the mother that it will be returned at discharge.

11. The orders are to give warfarin (Coumadin) 12.5 mg. On hand are 5 mg tablets. How many tablets would the nurse give the client?

1 0.5 tablet.
2 2 tablets.
3 2.5 tablets.
4 3 tablets.

12. A common test used to determine fetal status in the presence of pre-eclampsia is the nonstress test (NST). If this test is "reactive," the nurse knows that it means

1 The test was normal, showing an increased fetal heart rate (FHR) with fetal movement.
2 The test was normal, showing no change in FHR with fetal movement.
3 The test was abnormal, indicating a need for an immediate Oxytocin Challenge Test (OCT).
4 Ultrasound is indicated to determine fetal habitat and placental placement.

13. During a routine physical examination, the following reflexes are noted in a 9-month-old child. Which of the following is an abnormal finding?

1 Parachute reflex.
2 Neck righting reflex.
3 Rooting and sucking reflex.
4 Moro reflex.

14. A 40-year-old client is to be discharged and she wishes to walk outside. The nurse explains that the reason clients are discharged in a wheelchair is for

1 Comfort.
2 Convenience.
3 Safety.
4 Rehabilitation.

15. To perform the skill, "turning to the side-lying position," the nurse would lower the head of the bed, elevate the bed to working height,

move the client to the nurse's side of the bed, and flex the client's knees. The next intervention would be to

1   Roll the client on his side.
2   Reposition the client.
3   Place one hand on the client's hip and the other on his shoulder.
4   Reposition the client's arms so they are not under his body.

16.   When a client experiences a severe anaphylactic reaction to a medication, the nurse's initial action is to

1   Start an IV.
2   Assess vital signs.
3   Place the client in a supine position.
4   Prepare equipment for intubation.

17.   Instructing a client who has just received orders for nitroglycerin, the nurse informs the client that it should be taken

1   Every 2 to 3 hours during the day.
2   Before every meal and at bedtime.
3   At the first indication of chest pain.
4   Only when chest pain is not relieved by rest.

18.   A teenager comes into the nurse's office in a high school during lunch period and just hangs around. She states she might want to be a nurse some day. She says, "Nurses can help people when they feel bad." The best nursing response is

1   "Do you feel bad?"
2   "Is there some reason you've come in to see me?"
3   "You've been feeling 'bad'? Sit down and we'll talk."
4   "Yes, nurses can be helpful. I am glad you're interested in becoming a nurse."

19.   For a client in a long leg cast, which nursing intervention should receive the highest priority?

1   Handle the cast with the palms of the hands.
2   Keep the cast uncovered until it is dry.
3   Elevate the limb so the toes are higher than the hip.
4   Petal the cast edges with adhesive tape.

20.   The nurse has been teaching a client to use crutches. Which statement made by the client indicates a need for more teaching?

1   "I will not look down to watch my feet while I'm walking."
2   "I will place my weight on the hand grips."
3   "I will put my weak leg down first when going down stairs."
4   "I will raise the placement of the hand grips on the crutches as I get stronger."

21.   A nurse in her first trimester of pregnancy is working in the hospital. The nurse knows that she should avoid

1   Any client with an infection.
2   A 3-month-old infant with a generalized rash.
3   A child with a fever and upper respiratory disorder.
4   A client who has just been diagnosed with lupus erythematosus.

22.   The nurse collects the following information when taking a nursing history from a postmenopausal client. The data reveals a risk factor for the development of osteoporosis when the client

1   Has diabetes mellitus, Type II.
2   Has been on prednisone (Deltasone) for 3 months.
3   Swims laps in a pool, 3 times per week.
4   States she was never pregnant.

23.   In assessing an infant with pyloric stenosis, which one of the following clinical manifestations would be present?

1   Palpable olive-size mass in the lower abdomen.

2 Visible peristaltic waves passing left to right during and after feeding.

3 Severe projectile vomiting one hour after each feeding.

4 Fluid overload, demonstrated by bulging fontanels, widely separated cranial sutures, and urine specific gravity of 1.002.

24. The nurse is preparing a client for a myelogram using metrizamide (Amipaque), a water-soluble contrast material. The nurse will know the client understands the postmyelogram care regimen when she says

1 "I will need to keep my head elevated for at least 8 hours."

2 "I will need to lie flat for 12 to 24 hours."

3 "I will not be allowed to drink much liquid for 12 hours."

4 "I expect to have some itching and a stiff neck for a few days."

25. A client who is in respiratory failure requires endotracheal intubation and a ventilator. Nursing care while on the ventilator should include

1 Suctioning the endotracheal tube every 2 hours.

2 Encouraging the client to talk about his anxiety.

3 Keeping the endotracheal tube securely taped to the face.

4 Offering small sips of water as needed for oral comfort.

26. Nursing responsibility working on a psychiatric unit includes being able to recognize indications or signals of impending violent or assaultive behavior. This behavior could be

1 Foul language.

2 Hallucinations that are threatening, new, and commanding in nature.

3 Sudden withdrawal and refusal to speak.

4 Increased tendency to approach people and make physical contact, such as touching faces.

27. In teaching a newly diagnosed diabetic client about insulin self-injection, the nurse teaches that the injection site currently believed to be the best, because it provides the most rapid insulin absorption, is the

1 Arms.

2 Abdomen.

3 Thighs.

4 Buttocks.

28. The nurse, collecting data for a nursing history from a newly admitted client, learns that he has a Denver shunt. This suggests that he has a history of

1 Hydrocephalus.

2 Renal failure.

3 Peripheral occlusive disease.

4 Cirrhosis.

29. For a client with the diagnosis of acute pancreatitis, the nurse would include which critical component as part of the care plan?

1 Testing for Homan's sign.

2 Measuring the abdominal girth.

3 Performing a glucometer test.

4 Straining the urine.

30. To achieve the desired outcome of fracture healing, which nursing goal should receive the highest priority?

1 Maintain immobilization and alignment.

2 Provide optimal nutrition and hydration.

3 Promote independence in activities of daily living.

4 Provide relief from pain and discomfort.

31. An 8 year old with an acute asthma attack is admitted to the hospital. Initial nursing observations of the child will probably reveal

1 Noisy, hoarse inspirations.

2 Wheezing on expiration.

3 Labored abdominal breathing.

4 Flail chest with inspiratory wheeze.

32. A 34-year-old client is admitted with a diagnosis of hypoparathyroidism. One of the parameters the nurse will assess the client for is hypocalcemia. If present, the nurse would expect to observe

    1 Negative Chvostek's sign.
    2 Hyperventilation.
    3 Generalized edema.
    4 Spasms of hands and feet.

33. Following a missed abortion, a client has developed disseminated intravascular coagulation (DIC). The most critical nursing intervention for this client is to

    1 Administer ordered medications.
    2 Allay anxiety—provide emotional support.
    3 Administer ordered oxygen at 6 L/min.
    4 Encourage fluid intake.

34. A client brings her 1 year old to the well baby clinic. During the data collection, the nurse notes the presence of rib fractures. This condition suggests to the nurse she should look further for

    1 Osteoporosis.
    2 Child abuse.
    3 Cystic fibrosis.
    4 Malnutrition.

35. A client just received a diagnosis of carcinoma. While making morning rounds the day before surgery, the nurse observes the client crying. An appropriate response would be to

    1 Ignore the crying, as the nurse realizes the client may not want to talk.
    2 Acknowledge the client by saying, "Good morning," as the nurse passes the door and observe if she seems to wish to talk.
    3 Go in the room and ask her why she is crying.
    4 Go in the room, sit down, and stay quietly with her.

36. When auscultating the apical pulse of a client who has atrial fibrillation, the nurse would expect to hear a rhythm that is characterized by

    1 The presence of occasional coupled beats.
    2 Long pauses in an otherwise regular rhythm.
    3 A continuous and totally unpredictable irregularity.
    4 Slow but strong and regular beats.

37. When assessing pain in an infant, the nurse knows that infants typically display pain by

    1 Crying, increased appetite, and sleeping more.
    2 Withdrawing quietly and refusing to eat.
    3 Inconsolable crying, facial grimacing, and vigorous body movements.
    4 Increased sleeping time, refusal to eat, and irritability.

38. Which of the following blood chemistry results would the nurse expect to find elevated in a client with right-sided congestive heart failure?

    1 Ammonia.
    2 Albumin.
    3 LDH.
    4 CPK.

39. What should be the priority goal when a client assessment indicates the presence of a positive Homan's sign?

    1 Maintain a patent airway.
    2 Prevent infection.
    3 Foster fluid and electrolyte balance.
    4 Promote venous return.

40. When a toddler is hospitalized, the nurse knows that separation anxiety can be reduced by

    1 Having parents absent when painful procedures are performed.
    2 Not telling the toddler about upcoming painful experiences.

3 Setting limits and routines for parental visits.

4 Having parents present as much as possible, preparing for separations, and use of transitional objects ("Loveys").

41. A 75-year-old client has the diagnosis of organic brain syndrome (OBS). In planning the daily schedule, it is important for the nurse to understand that the client

1 May have moderate-to-severe memory impairment and short periods of concentration.

2 Will be more comfortable with a rigid daily schedule.

3 Is more likely to be able to remember current experiences than past ones.

4 Can usually be trusted to be responsible for her daily care needs.

42. A client with COPD has developed secondary polycythemia. Which nursing diagnosis would be included in the care plan because of the polycythemia?

1 Fluid volume deficit related to blood loss.

2 Impaired tissue perfusion related to thrombosis.

3 Activity intolerance related to dyspnea.

4 Risk for infection related to suppressed immune response.

43. Appropriate toys for a 3-month-old infant would include

1 Soft, colorful squeeze toys and teething toys.

2 Teething toys with small, removable parts.

3 Push and pull toys, and pounding toys.

4 Balls and toys that stimulate the senses.

44. The nurse is teaching a client with a new colostomy how to apply an appliance to a colostomy. How much skin should remain exposed between the stoma and the ring of the appliance?

1 1/8 inch.

2 1/2 inch.

3 3/4 inch.

4 1 inch.

45. A client's physician has suggested that a lecithin/sphingomyelin (L/S) ratio be done. The client is 34 weeks pregnant. The client is very nervous and asks the nurse why this test must be done. The best response is that this test

1 Will indicate the sex of the baby.

2 Determines the maturity of the baby's lungs.

3 Has diagnostic capability to ascertain if anything is wrong.

4 Detects neural tube defect.

46. A client was admitted with the diagnosis of antisocial behavior. He had beat up his girlfriend and was brought to the hospital for a court-ordered evaluation. During the nurse's interaction with the client, he asked where she lives, whom she dates, and other personal information. He said, "I just want to get to know you better. I like you. You're the only one I can really talk to." The best nursing response would be

1 "You're getting too involved with me. Maybe another nurse would be more appropriate for you."

2 "Let's talk about my purpose in working with you and your feelings about it."

3 "Why are you focusing on me all the time?"

4 "I think you're trying to avoid talking about you and your problems."

47. When caring for an unconscious child, the nurse's *primary* concern must always be

1 Airway protection and adequate respiratory status.

2 Decreasing intracranial pressure.

3 Fluid balance and cardiac stability.

4 Maintaining range of motion and muscle tone.

48. A hypothyroid client has orders for all of the following medications. The nurse would evaluate the client most closely following administration of which medication?

    1 Meperidine (Demerol).
    2 Ibuprofen (Motrin).
    3 Levothyroxine (Synthroid).
    4 Digoxin (Lanoxin).

49. A client has been receiving chemotherapy for the treatment of breast cancer. She is now to start receiving daily injections of filgrastim (Neupogen). The nurse would assess for a therapeutic response to this drug by monitoring which laboratory test result?

    1 Blood urea nitrogen (BUN).
    2 Potassium.
    3 Platelets.
    4 White blood cell count (WBC).

50. A nurse is in the situation of an emergency delivery and, as the baby's head is born, observes the cord draped around the baby's neck. The nursing action is to

    1 Wait until the placenta is delivered to prevent damage.
    2 Gently push the baby's head back in to release pressure.
    3 Cut the cord to prevent damage to the baby.
    4 Slip the cord over the baby's head to prevent circulatory impairment.

51. A client is to receive 65 mg of gentamycin (Garamycin). Available is a solution containing 80 mg per 2 mL. How much of this solution should the nurse draw up?

    1 0.6 mL.
    2 1.2 mL.
    3 1.6 mL.
    4 2.5 mL.

52. The laboratory result that should be monitored regularly in a client who is receiving gentamycin (Garamycin) is

    1 Serum creatinine.
    2 Serum calcium.
    3 Platelets.
    4 White blood cell count (WBC).

53. When assessing a child suspected of having epiglottitis, the nursing action is to

    1 Lay the child down flat to calm him/her down.
    2 Give IM antibiotics as standard orders while attempting to start an IV.
    3 Keep the child calm while administering 100% oxygen and awaiting an expert at intubation.
    4 Send the child to x-ray immediately for a chest x-ray.

54. The nurse finds a manipulative client in the TV room at midnight watching an old movie. The nurse reminds him that the TV set is to be shut off at 12:30 AM. He ignores her. When the nurse returns 30 minutes later, he tells her not to turn off the TV because he is just starting another movie and he intends to watch it. The best nursing response is

    1 "OK, but that's it after this one!"
    2 "No one else is allowed to watch TV this late."
    3 "Apparently there is some confusion about the rules."
    4 "You are aware of the TV rule and I'm turning off the TV now."

55. A nursing mother has developed mastitis and has symptoms of chills, 103°F temperature, and elevated pulse. The nurse, making a home visit, should include instructions to

    1 Leave the breast free of support or binding brassiere.
    2 Apply heat to the breast.

3 Continue to breast-feed as necessary.

4 Empty the breast every 4 hours regardless of infant's feeding schedule.

56. A client's laboratory results indicate a creatinine level of 7 mg/dL. This finding would lead the nurse to place the highest priority on monitoring the client's

1 Temperature.
2 Intake and output.
3 Capillary refill.
4 Pupillary reflex.

57. A client with a bile duct obstruction is jaundiced. Which intervention will be most effective in controlling the itching associated with his jaundice?

1 Be sure the client's nails are clean and short.
2 Maintain the room temperature at 72° to 75° F.
3 Provide tepid water for bathing.
4 Use alcohol for back rubs.

58. When using nasotracheal suction to clear a client's airway of excessive secretions, the nurse would

1 Lubricate the catheter with sterile petrolatum.
2 Insert the catheter with a finger on the vent.
3 Place a finger over the vent intermittently while withdrawing the catheter.
4 Limit any attempts at suctioning to 30 seconds or less.

59. A client's hemoglobin is 10 gm/dL and the hematocrit is 30 percent. Based on these lab results, the highest priority nursing goal would be to

1 Promote skin integrity.
2 Conserve the client's energy.
3 Prevent constipation.
4 Encourage mobility.

60. The nurse working in a prenatal clinic has been advised that the physician should immediately see any client who presents with

1 Heartburn.
2 Diastolic blood pressure over 85.
3 Ankle edema.
4 Blurred vision.

61. A client with a history of pernicious anemia has been admitted to a long-term care facility. There are no orders written. The LVN would ask the charge nurse to question the physician about obtaining medical orders for

1 Folic acid.
2 Iron.
3 Vitamin B_6.
4 Vitamin B_{12}.

62. When a child is admitted with the diagnosis of croup, why are cool mist vaporizers better to use than hot steam vaporizers?

1 The temperature of the mist is irrelevant because the child needs humidity.
2 More moisture can be delivered in cool mist than with hot steam.
3 Small children are more resistant to anything that is hot.
4 The cool mist relieves swelling in the airways and makes breathing easier.

63. A client has been receiving digoxin (Lanoxin) 0.125 mg daily for a week. When the nurse visits him at home, the client tells the nurse about several problems that have been developing over the last few days. Which of these complaints is suggestive of digoxin toxicity?

1 Constipation.
2 Urinary frequency.
3 Loss of appetite.
4 Ankle edema.

64. A client with chronic renal failure is on continuous ambulatory peritoneal dialysis (CAPD).

Which nursing diagnosis would have the highest priority?

1   Powerlessness.
2   High risk for infection.
3   Altered nutrition: less than body requirements.
4   High risk for fluid volume deficit.

65.   A 42-year-old housewife is admitted to the psychiatric unit. She worries about staying clean on the unit and refuses to sit on the chairs or use the eating utensils. She is constantly washing her hands "to get the germs off." She is pleasant to approach, follows simple directions, but becomes upset when her ritual is interrupted. Her diagnosis is obsessive-compulsive disorder. While attempting to decrease her anxiety, which of the following nursing responses would be most therapeutic?

1   "This is a hospital and I can assure you we keep it clean."
2   "If you continue washing your hands, you are going to have skin problems."
3   "What can I do to help?"
4   "You seem uncomfortable right now. When you finish washing your hands, let's take a walk around the unit."

66.   A type I diabetic client tells the nurse she doesn't like what is on her dinner tray and refuses to eat it. The best intervention is to

1   Call the physician for a different diet order.
2   Obtain a regular diet tray from the kitchen and remove all sugar and desserts.
3   Order a sandwich and soup from the kitchen and make a referral to the dietician.
4   Ask the kitchen staff to send another diabetic meal tray for the client.

67.   The charge nurse instructs the LVN to admit a new client from the ER because all of the RNs are busy. The most appropriate response is

1   "I will be happy to help out; I know everyone is busy."
2   "I will put the client in bed and orient him to the environment only."
3   "I'm sorry, I can't help you because my license doesn't allow me to admit clients."
4   "I will admit the client but I will need to document that I'm working outside my license parameters in case there is a problem."

68.   When completing the preop check list, the client asks the nurse, "What exactly am I going to have done in surgery?" The appropriate response is

1   To explain the procedure in nonmedical terms to the client.
2   Ask the client what the physician explained to him.
3   Check the chart to see what the physician explained and repeat the information to him.
4   Explain that you don't know and he should ask the physician when he sees him before surgery.

69.   A client in hepatic coma has orders for lactulose to reduce blood ammonia. The nurse would know that the medication is working when

1   Watery diarrhea occurs.
2   The client has 2 to 3 stools/day.
3   The client is constipated.
4   Dehydration occurs and can be observed in the client's skin condition.

70.   A physician has written orders to test nasogastric drainage every hour for a client on mechanical ventilation. The nurse recognizes the importance of this action because

1   The NG tube may become dislodged.
2   The pH should be maintained below 5.
3   Stress ulcers are frequently associated with mechanical ventilation.
4   It will determine if the antacids are working.

71. The nurse is to assess the capillary refill time of a client who has a leg cast. When the nurse compresses one of the client's toenails and releases the compression, the nurse would expect the color to return to the nail within

    1   1 second.
    2   3 seconds.
    3   10 seconds.
    4   15 seconds.

72. While administering an enema to a client, the nurse will position the container

    1   No more than 18 inches above the rectum.
    2   Three to 4 inches above the rectum.
    3   As high as the client can tolerate.
    4   Three feet above bed level.

73. The nurse responsible for planning an elderly, senile client's schedule knows that it is most important that the daily activities

    1   Are changed each day to meet the need for variety.
    2   Provide many opportunities for making choices to stimulate involvement and interest.
    3   Are highly structured to reduce anxiety.
    4   Involve physically limited activity, as the client tires easily.

74. While caring for a client who had a left leg above-the-knee amputation several days earlier, the client cheerfully begins talking about getting back to the "old tennis courts" for a "set or two." His emotional acceptance of this condition can be interpreted as

    1   Denying his altered body image.
    2   Adjusting well to his altered mobility.
    3   Accepting his loss.
    4   Beginning to deal with his limitations.

75. Following an angry outburst the previous evening, a client says, "I'm feeling calmer now. I don't know what got into me. You all must think I'm crazy." The best response to this statement would be

    1   "That's all right. We're here to help you."
    2   "Why would you think that?"
    3   "You think your behavior was crazy?"
    4   "How were you feeling last evening?"

76. The symptom the nurse would observe for as a cardinal sign of eclampsia during pregnancy is

    1   Weight gain of 1 to 2 pounds a week.
    2   Concentrated urine.
    3   Hypertension.
    4   Lassitude and fatigue.

77. The nurse is assigned to work with a client diagnosed as having pernicious anemia. In evaluating the diet for the client, the nurse would know the client understands dietary parameters when he chooses

    1   Meat, milk, cheese.
    2   Whole grains, cereals.
    3   Fruits, green leafy vegetables.
    4   Organ meats, yellow vegetables.

78. After application of a leg cast following a fracture, the client is unable to feel pressure on his toes and complains of tingling. These signs indicate

    1   Pressure on a nerve.
    2   Phantom pain syndrome.
    3   Overmedication with an analgesic.
    4   Improper alignment of the fracture.

79. The client paces the floor, wringing her hands saying, "Something is going to happen. Help me! Help me!" The nurse says, "You look very upset." The nurse is using the technique of

    1   Giving feedback.
    2   Being reassuring.
    3   Validating a nonverbal observation.
    4   Seeking clarification.

80. A client brings her 1 year old to the well baby clinic. During the assessment, the nurse notes the presence of rib fractures. This condition suggests to the nurse she should further assess for

1   Osteoporosis.
2   Child abuse.
3   Cystic fibrosis.
4   Malnutrition.

81. A client on the oncology unit is in a great deal of pain but it is controlled with PCA—patient-controlled IV analgesia. The nurse explains to the client's family that the rationale for using this method is that it

1   Allows nurses to care for more clients.
2   Enables clients to administer medication when pain is experienced.
3   Results in less pain medication used by client.
4   Programs medication dosages to remain within acceptable limits.

82. When evaluating the client's understanding of a low potassium diet, the nurse will know he understands if he says that he will avoid

1   Pasta.
2   Raw apples.
3   Dry cereal.
4   French bread.

83. Urecholine (bethanechol chloride) is ordered PRN for a client following a transurethral resection (TUR). Which of the following conditions would need to be present for the nurse to administer this drug?

1   Complaints of bladder spasms.
2   Complaints of severe pain.
3   Inability to void.
4   Frequent episodes of painful urination.

84. The milliliters of drug that should be used to give 0.5 gm if the label on the bottle reads 5 gm in 10 mL is

1   2.0 mL.
2   1.0 mL.
3   0.5 mL.
4   5.0 mL.

85. After removing the fecal impaction, the client complains of feeling light-headed and the pulse rate is 44. The priority intervention is to

1   Monitor vital signs.
2   Place in shock position.
3   Call the physician.
4   Begin CPR.

86. A 4 year old child with celiac disease is admitted to the hospital with abdominal pain, distention and vomiting. Intussusception is the suspected diagnosis. The nurse, in completing data collection, will ask the parents if the symptoms

1   Occurred suddenly.
2   Developed over the last few days.
3   Were mild, but bothersome.
4   Were preceded by the ingestion of certain foods.

87. Which nursing action is the most critical when caring for a client who is receiving continuous nasogastric tube feedings?

1   Warming the feeding to room temperature.
2   Maintaining accurate records of intake and output.
3   Flushing the tube with water every 4 hours.
4   Keeping the client in a semi-Fowler's position.

88. Following a cesarean section, paralytic ileus may be a complication. According to the physician's orders, an important assessment would be to

1   Administer PO fluids only.

2 Insert a nasogastric tube.
3 Listen for bowel sounds.
4 Insert a rectal tube.

89. A client with thrombophlebitis should be positioned so that his legs are

1 Dependent.
2 Flat on the bed.
3 Elevated about 30 degrees.
4 Elevated about 60 degrees.

90. A client has reported to the ambulatory surgical center for a hernia repair. While in the preoperative area, the client tells the nurse he is very nervous about the surgery. The best response by the nurse is

1 "What did the physician tell you she is planning to do?"
2 "Do you usually get nervous about new experiences?"
3 "Your physician is very competent and will help you get better."
4 "Tell me how you are feeling right now."

COMPREHENSIVE TEST 3

Answers with Rationale

1. (3) Protamine sulfate is the antagonist for Heparin. Answer (2), vitamin K, is the antagonist for Coumadin. Answer (4) is the antagonist for magnesium sulfate.

> *Nursing Process:* Planning
> *Client Needs:* Safe, Effective Care Environment
> *Clinical Area:* Medical Nursing

2. (4) Closed chest drainage is used for lobectomies to re-establish negative pressure in the chest. Because the breathing mechanism operates on the principle of negative pressure, this is an essential action. The other interventions would follow this one.

> *Nursing Process:* Implementation
> *Client Needs:* Safe, Effective Care Environment
> *Clinical Area:* Surgical Nursing

3. (4) By first removing the old patch, the risk of overdosing the client is minimized. The skin should not be wiped with alcohol and the patch should be applied without rubbing. Patches may be placed under clothing or on exposed skin.

> *Nursing Process:* Implementation
> *Client Needs:* Safe, Effective Care Environment
> *Clinical Area:* Medical Nursing

4. (1) A full course of antibiotics is necessary to destroy the causative organism. Any change in neurological status could be a developing CNS infection (e.g., meningitis). Children usually feel able to return to school after 24 to 48 hours of antibiotics, and will self-limit their own activity. Avoiding dental hygiene is not advised nor helpful in preventing otitis media.

> *Nursing Process:* Implementation
> *Client Needs:* Health Promotion and Maintenance
> *Clinical Area:* Pediatric Nursing

5. (4) It is best to plan any activity, particularly therapy, to follow the compulsive activity because anxiety is lowest at this time.

> *Nursing Process:* Planning
> *Client Needs:* Psychosocial Integrity
> *Clinical Area:* Psychiatric Nursing

6. (3) The first action is to move the client to his left side and lower the head of the bed. In this position air will rise to the right atrium. The charge nurse should then be notified.

> *Nursing Process:* Implementation
> *Client Needs:* Safe, Effective Care Environment
> *Clinical Area:* Medical Nursing

7. (3) A regular nipple is too hard and will make it difficult for the infant to suck, causing unnecessary fatigue. A premie soft nipple should be used.

> *Nursing Process:* Planning
> *Client Needs:* Safe, Effective Care Environment
> *Clinical Area:* Maternity Nursing

8. (4) The appropriate intervention is to withhold the thiazide medication until the nurse receives further orders and report K^+ level to the physician. Normal K^+ is 3.5 to 5.5 mEq/l.

His NA⁺ level is normal (range 135 to 145 mEq/l).

Nursing Process: Evaluation
Client Needs: Safe, Effective Care Environment
Clinical Area: Medical Nursing

9. (2) Blind clients become anxious when they hear someone enter the room without talking.

Nursing Process: Planning
Client Needs: Psychosocial Integrity
Clinical Area: Medical Nursing

10. (1) In some cultures, garlic is worn to protect against illness. Asking the mother to explain will provide data that can be used to assess whether this is part of a culture-based health practice. If so, it is important to take into account when the health team is formulating a client care plan.

Nursing Process: Implementation
Client Needs: Psychosocial Integrity
Clinical Area: Pediatric Nursing

11. (3) This computation can be done using the formula D (dose desired) divided by H (dose on hand) multiplied by Q (quantity of dose on hand). 12.5 divided by 5 multiplied by 1 equals 2.5 tablets.

Nursing Process: Planning
Client Needs: Safe, Effective Care Environment
Clinical Area: Medical Nursing

12. (1) Reactive = good outcome. Increased FHR with movement indicates normal reaction and adequate CNS integration.

Nursing Process: Data Collection
Client Needs: Physiological Integrity
Clinical Area: Maternity Nursing

13. (4) The Moro reflex begins to fade at the third or fourth month. Thus, if found in a nine month old, it would be abnormal. The remaining reflexes would be normal development.

Nursing Process: Data Collection
Client Needs: Safe, Effective Care Environment
Clinical Area: Pediatric Nursing

14. (3) Transportation by wheelchair can prevent falls and injury; therefore, safety is the important issue.

Nursing Process: Implementation
Client Needs: Safe, Effective Care Environment
Clinical Area: Medical Nursing

15. (3) Before rolling the client on his side, the nurse's hands must be in the correct position to turn. Answer (4) would be the final intervention.

Nursing Process: Implementation
Client Needs: Safe, Effective Care Environment
Clinical Area: Medical Nursing

16. (3) The shock position is necessary to maintain vital signs. The other interventions may be carried out, but are not initial actions.

Nursing Process: Implementation
Client Needs: Physiological Integrity
Clinical Area: Medical Nursing

17. (3) Nitroglycerin should be taken whenever the client feels a full, pressure feeling or tightness in his or her chest, and not wait until chest pain is severe. It can also be taken prophylactically to prevent an anginal attack before engaging in an activity known to cause angina.

Nursing Process: Implementation
Client Needs: Health Promotion and
Maintenance
Clinical Area: Medical Nursing

18. (3) The nurse is responding to the unspoken communication she is hearing. This response opens up communication and provides the opportunity for the teenager to talk about feeling bad. (1) and (2) ask for a "yes or no" response which would not facilitate communication, and (4) is a tangential response.

Nursing Process: Data Collection
Client Needs: Psychosocial Integrity
Clinical Area: Psychiatric Nursing

19. (3) Although all of the interventions are appropriate in the care of a client with a casted limb, it is most critical to maintain limb elevation. This nursing action prevents edema which could compress blood vessels and nerves.

Nursing Process: Implementation
Client Needs: Safe, Effective Care
Environment
Clinical Area: Surgical Nursing

20. (4) The hand grips should be placed so that the elbows are flexed at 20 to 30 degrees when standing with the crutches. This placement should not be changed as long as the client continues to need crutches. The other statements indicate effective learning.

Nursing Process: Evaluation
Client Needs: Health Promotion and
Maintenance
Clinical Area: Medical Nursing

21. (2) German measles or rubella, if contracted in the first trimester of pregnancy, may result in a child with congenital malformations of the heart, eye and ear, as well as mental retardation.

Nursing Process: Planning
Client Needs: Health Promotion and
Maintenance
Clinical Area: Maternity Nursing

22. (2) Glucocorticoids, such as prednisone, promote protein catabolism and are a known risk factor for the development of osteoporosis. Swimming would be an exercise to reduce risk of osteoporosis.

Nursing Process: Data Collection
Client Needs: Physiological Integrity
Clinical Area: Medical Nursing

23. (2) Peristaltic waves pass left to right with this condition. Pyloric stenosis presents in early infancy with projectile vomiting right after feeding. Dehydration and electrolyte imbalances are possible complications if therapy is not performed; thus, fluid overload is not a symptom. A small mass may be found in the upper right quadrant.

Nursing Process: Data Collection
Client Needs: Safe, Effective Care
Environment
Clinical Area: Pediatric Nursing

24. (1) The head must be kept elevated because this drug could provoke a seizure if it reaches the brain in a bolus form. After myelography that uses an oil-based contrast medium (Pantopaque), clients are kept flat. Forcing fluids helps prevent postmyelogram headache by replacing lost spinal fluid. Itching suggests an allergic reaction, while a stiff neck suggests meningeal irritation; neither is an expected response to a myelogram.

Nursing Process: Evaluation
Client Needs: Health Promotion and
Maintenance
Clinical Area: Surgical Nursing

25. (3) The endotracheal tube must be kept in place because it is the conduit between the ventilator and the client's lungs. Also, accidental extubation can produce laryngospasm. Suctioning is done only as needed, rather than on a fixed schedule. An intubated client cannot speak or swallow safely.

> *Nursing Process:* Planning
> *Client Needs:* Safe, Effective Care Environment
> *Clinical Area:* Medical Nursing

26. (2) Violent behavior often occurs as a response to a real or imagined threat. Hallucinations can be threatening in nature. Foul language may or may not be an indication of impending violence. Threatening hallucinations are more predictive of possible acting out behavior.

> *Nursing Process:* Data Collection
> *Client Needs:* Psychosocial Integrity
> *Clinical Area:* Psychiatric Nursing

27. (2) Studies have shown that insulin is most rapidly and consistently absorbed from the subcutaneous tissue of the abdomen. The current thinking, therefore, is that insulin injections should be rotated among sites on the abdomen alone (with the exception of 1 inch around the umbilicus), rather than among the other available anatomic sites, i.e., arms, thighs and buttocks.

> *Nursing Process:* Planning
> *Client Needs:* Health Promotion and Maintenance
> *Clinical Area:* Medical Nursing

28. (4) The Denver shunt is a type of peritoneovascular shunt used in the treatment of clients who have cirrhosis with ascites. The shunt diverts ascitic fluid from the abdomen into the jugular vein or the vena cava.

> *Nursing Process:* Data Collection
> *Client Needs:* Physiological Integrity
> *Clinical Area:* Medical Nursing

29. (3) Hyperglycemia is a common finding in acute pancreatitis because the islet cells may not be able to produce adequate amounts of insulin. An important component of the treatment is to administer regular insulin to treat the hyperglycemia.

> *Nursing Process:* Planning
> *Client Needs:* Physiological Integrity
> *Clinical Area:* Medical Nursing

30. (1) Maintaining the prescribed immobilization and body alignment will keep the fracture fragments in close anatomical proximity, thereby promoting functional fracture healing. This goal should receive the highest priority. The other goals, although applicable in the care of a client with a fracture, do not have as high a priority in meeting this particular desired outcome.

> *Nursing Process:* Planning
> *Client Needs:* Safe, Effective Care Environment
> *Clinical Area:* Surgical Nursing

31. (2) The hallmark of asthma is wheezing. Wheezing is an expiratory sound. There is no vocal cord involvement so "hoarse" is unlikely. Abdominal breathing does not occur with asthma.

> *Nursing Process:* Data Collection
> *Client Needs:* Physiological Integrity
> *Clinical Area:* Pediatric Nursing

32. (4) Calcium produces a sedative effect on nerve cells and is essential for the transmission of nerve impulses. A deficit of calcium produces abnormal muscle contractions and is manifested by carpopedal spasms. Acute muscular spasms (tetany) may be potentially fatal.

The Chvostek's sign would be positive if hypocalcemia is present. Edema or hyperventilation would not be noted with this diagnosis.

> *Nursing Process:* Data Collection
> *Client Needs:* Physiological Integrity
> *Clinical Area:* Medical Nursing

33. (1) In DIC, the client begins to hemorrhage after the initial hypercoagulability uses up the clotting factors in the blood. Administering heparin, therefore, is a critical nursing intervention. Heparin prevents clot formation and increases available fibrinogen, coagulation factors, and platelets. The other actions have lesser priority. Oxygen would be administered at 2 to 3 L/min.

> *Nursing Process:* Implementation
> *Client Needs:* Safe, Effective Care Environment
> *Clinical Area:* Maternity Nursing

34. (2) The bones of a 1-year-old child are flexible and unlikely to break unless subjected to unusual stress. This could occur through child abuse; the nurse is legally responsible to report any case of suspected child abuse.

> *Nursing Process:* Data Collection
> *Client Needs:* Safe, Effective Care Environment
> *Clinical Area:* Pediatric Nursing

35. (4) The most effective communication technique in this case would be silence; support the client nonverbally, accept her, and open up the opportunity for an expression of feelings.

> *Nursing Process:* Implementation
> *Client Needs:* Psychosocial Integrity
> *Clinical Area:* Psychiatric Nursing

36. (3) In atrial fibrillation, multiple ectopic foci stimulate the atria to contract. The AV node is unable to transmit all of these impulses to the ventricles, resulting in a pattern of highly irregular ventricular contractions.

> *Nursing Process:* Data Collection
> *Client Needs:* Physiological Integrity
> *Clinical Area:* Medical Nursing

37. (3) Facial grimacing, inconsolable crying, and flailing body movements have been described as diagnostic signs of pain in infants (data from CHEOPS Scale). Changes in appetite and sleep can be attributed to other causes.

> *Nursing Process:* Data Collection
> *Client Needs:* Psychosocial Integrity
> *Clinical Area:* Pediatric Nursing

38. (3) The liver becomes engorged with blood in right-sided congestive heart failure. Liver function studies, such as the LDH, an enzyme production test for the liver, will be abnormally elevated in 40 percent of the clients. Serum bilirubin is also frequently increased. Ammonia and albumin, also liver tests, will not be elevated.

> *Nursing Process:* Evaluation
> *Client Needs:* Physiological Integrity
> *Clinical Area:* Medical Nursing

39. (4) A positive Homan's sign may indicate the presence of thrombophlebitis; therefore, promoting venous return is the priority nursing goal. The other goals are not relevant to this assessment finding.

> *Nursing Process:* Planning
> *Client Needs:* Safe, Effective Care Environment
> *Clinical Area:* Medical Nursing

40. (4) Parents and transitional objects have been shown in research to decrease anxiety. Having parents present as much as possible, especially for painful procedures, helps de-

crease anxiety. Explaining upcoming procedures in language the toddler can understand will also help decrease their anxiety.

Nursing Process: Planning
Client Needs: Psychosocial Integrity
Clinical Area: Pediatric Nursing

41. (1) It is important to remember that OBS clients usually have some memory and concentration impairment. The degree depends upon the individual and is influenced by the basic personality structure and the cause of the problem.

Nursing Process: Planning
Client Needs: Psychosocial Integrity
Clinical Area: Psychiatric Nursing

42. (2) Chronic hypoxia associated with COPD may stimulate excessive RBC production (polycythemia). This results in increased blood viscosity and the risk of thrombosis. The other nursing diagnoses are not applicable in this situation.

Nursing Process: Planning
Client Needs: Physiological Integrity
Clinical Area: Medical Nursing

43. (1) Toys should be visually appealing without small parts which could choke an infant. Exploration through the mouth begins at 3 months. Push and pull toys and balls are appropriate for the mobile, older baby.

Nursing Process: Planning
Client Needs: Psychosocial Integrity
Clinical Area: Pediatric Nursing

44. (1) A colostomy appliance should be cut to fit the stoma so that there is no pressure placed on the stoma by the appliance and there is a minimum amount of skin exposed to fecal drainage. Leaving 1/8 inch of skin exposed conforms to these criteria.

Nursing Process: Implementation
Client Needs: Health Promotion and Maintenance
Clinical Area: Surgical Nursing

45. (2) This test examines amniotic fluid for the presence of surfactant to determine fetal lung maturity. When lecithin is two or more times greater than sphingomyelin, the infant is unlikely to develop respiratory distress syndrome. This ratio usually occurs at the 35th week of pregnancy. An amniocentesis test will determine the sex of the baby and whether there is a problem such as Down's syndrome.

Nursing Process: Evaluation
Client Needs: Health Promotion and Maintenance
Clinical Area: Maternity Nursing

46. (2) The nurse is structuring the relationship and giving the client an opening to talk about his feelings. She is also refocusing the communication. (1) is incorrect because the nurse is avoiding the issue of the client's feelings. (2) is incorrect because it asks him to analyze and give a reason for his behavior. The focus needs to be on his feelings and behaviors. (4) is incorrect because it is a judgmental statement and may put the client on the defensive.

Nursing Process: Implementation
Client Needs: Psychosocial Integrity
Clinical Area: Psychiatric Nursing

47. (1) As neuro status deteriorates, the airway *must* be assured to avoid compromising oxygenation or aspiration. Hypoxia will exacerbate brain injury. The other answers are appropriate goals *after* airway patency is assured.

Nursing Process: Planning
Client Needs: Safe, Effective Care Environment
Clinical Area: Pediatric Nursing

48. (1) Hypothyroidism reduces the metabolic rate and prolongs the sedative effects of medications. Narcotics, such as meperidine, are especially dangerous and should be given in smaller doses. The client must be closely monitored for signs of oversedation and respiratory depression.

   Nursing Process: Evaluation
   Client Needs: Safe, Effective Care Environment
   Clinical Area: Medical Nursing

49. (4) Filgrastim stimulates the production of WBCs. It is given to clients experiencing bone marrow depression with leukopenia secondary to cancer chemotherapy.

   Nursing Process: Evaluation
   Client Needs: Physiological Integrity
   Clinical Area: Medical Nursing

50. (4) The nursing action is to gently slip the cord (which is fairly elastic) over the baby's head. The nurse would never wait until the placenta is delivered, as the infant could become hypoxic. The nurse could not push the baby's head back in. The cord should not be cut at this time to prevent hypoxia.

   Nursing Process: Implementation
   Client Needs: Safe, Effective Care Environment
   Clinical Area: Maternity Nursing

51. (3) This computation can be done using the formula of D (dose desired) divided by H (dose on hand) multiplied by V (volume). 65 divided by 80 multiplied by 2 equals 1.625 mL.

   Nursing Process: Implementation
   Client Needs: Safe, Effective Care Environment
   Clinical Area: Medical Nursing

52. (1) Gentamycin, a potent aminoglycoside antibiotic, has the potential for causing nephrotoxicity. Renal function studies such as the serum creatinine and BUN should be monitored regularly to detect impaired renal function.

   Nursing Process: Evaluation
   Client Needs: Safe, Effective Care Environment
   Clinical Area: Medical Nursing

53. (3) Keeping the child calm is important because any added trauma to the airway, even from crying, could cause airway obstruction. Children should be positioned upright in "sniffing position" to help maintain airway patency. Oxygen is delivered in the method best tolerated by the child and only the most experienced nurse should attempt intubation—difficult because of swollen tissues. Children suspected of having epiglottitis should *never* be left alone.

   Nursing Process: Implementation
   Client Needs: Safe, Effective Care Environment
   Clinical Area: Pediatric Nursing

54. (4) The nurse is setting clear limits on the client's behavior. He is testing her to see if she will follow through on what she said she would do. (1) is incorrect. She is allowing the client to manipulate her which will reinforce his noncompliance. (2) and (3) are also incorrect. The nurse is not addressing the real issue and she is opening up the subject for negotiation rather than setting clear limits.

   Nursing Process: Implementation
   Client Needs: Psychosocial Integrity
   Clinical Area: Psychiatric Nursing

55. (2) The most effective nursing action is local application of heat to the breast. Other treatment will include antibiotics and analgesics for pain. This mother needs a snug-fitting,

supportive brassiere. Breast-feeding may or may not be continued; if not, the breast should be emptied every 4 hours to prevent engorgement.

Nursing Process: Planning
Client Needs: Physiological Integrity
Clinical Area: Maternity Nursing

56. (2) This elevated creatinine suggests impaired renal function. Monitoring intake and output will provide data related to renal function. The other findings would not be indicative of renal function.

Nursing Process: Data Collection
Client Needs: Safe, Effective Care Environment
Clinical Area: Medical Nursing

57. (3) Itching is made worse by vasodilation. Tepid water prevents excessive vasodilation. Warm environmental temperatures promote vasodilation. Alcohol not only produces vasodilation, but is drying to the skin which further compounds the problem of itching. Keeping the nails clean and short will help prevent skin irritation and infection if the client scratches, but will not prevent the itching from occurring.

Nursing Process: Planning
Client Needs: Physiological Integrity
Clinical Area: Medical Nursing

58. (3) To prevent trauma to the mucous membranes lining the airway, suction should be applied only while withdrawing the catheter. The catheter should be lubricated with a water-soluble substance to prevent lipoidal pneumonia. Suctioning attempts should be limited to 10 seconds to prevent hypoxia.

Nursing Process: Implementation
Client Needs: Safe, Effective Care Environment
Clinical Area: Medical Nursing

59. (2) These test results indicate anemia. Impaired oxygen carrying capacity of red blood cells causes cellular hypoxia and results in fatigue. Conserving energy limits oxygen expenditure and minimizes fatigue. Increased mobility increases the demand for oxygen and contributes to fatigue. Although hypoxic tissues are more vulnerable to breakdown, protecting the integumentary system is not as high a priority as is the promotion of overall oxygenation. Constipation is not a problem in anemia.

Nursing Process: Planning
Client Needs: Physiological Integrity
Clinical Area: Medical Nursing

60. (4) Blurred vision is an advanced indicator of pregnancy-induced hypertension (PIH) and the physician should see the client immediately.

Nursing Process: Planning
Client Needs: Physiological Integrity
Clinical Area: Maternity Nursing

61. (4) In pernicious anemia, a person cannot absorb vitamin B_{12} because of a deficiency of the intrinsic factor. The person must regularly receive vitamin B_{12} parenterally to prevent neurologic deficits. The other listed nutrients are not effective in the treatment of pernicious anemia.

Nursing Process: Planning
Client Needs: Physiological Integrity
Clinical Area: Medical Nursing

62. (4) Swollen, irritated tissues will vasoconstrict and swelling is reduced in response to cold and humidity. Humidity also helps loosen secretions. While amounts of moisture delivered may vary, the vasoconstriction offered by cold mist is most beneficial.

Nursing Process: Planning
Client Needs: Physiological Integrity
Clinical Area: Pediatric Nursing

63. (3) Anorexia is a common, and early, manifestation of digoxin toxicity. The other complaints are not related to digoxin.

> *Nursing Process:* Evaluation
> *Client Needs:* Physiological Integrity
> *Clinical Area:* Medical Nursing

64. (2) There is a high risk of infection in clients receiving CAPD because microorganisms can enter the body by migrating around, or through, the peritoneal dialysis catheter. They may also enter through contaminated dialysate solutions. The other diagnoses are not life threatening for a client on CAPD.

> *Nursing Process:* Planning
> *Client Needs:* Physiological Integrity
> *Clinical Area:* Medical Nursing

65. (4) This nursing response acknowledges the client's feelings and allows her to complete her ritual. This decreases her anxiety. The walk will help to decrease some of the anxious energy, as well as showing her that the nurse is interested in her.

> *Nursing Process:* Planning
> *Client Needs:* Psychosocial Integrity
> *Clinical Area:* Psychiatric Nursing

66. (4) The client must have the correct carbohydrates, fats and proteins determined by the specific diet plan so a new tray should come from the kitchen. Substituting food may not provide the correct balance.

> *Nursing Process:* Implementation
> *Client Needs:* Physiological Integrity
> *Clinical Area:* Medical Nursing

67. (2) Licensed vocational/practical nurses can only assist in the admission of clients. They can orient the client to the environment, take vital signs, and weigh clients. They do not make initial assessments or develop care plans.

> *Nursing Process:* Implementation
> *Client Needs:* Safe, Effective Care Environment
> *Clinical Area:* Medical Nursing

68. (2) Find out exactly what the client has been told. Many times they have been given an explanation and only need further clarification. If the client does not have an adequate understanding of the procedure, have the charge nurse notify the physician that he needs to see the client. The physician has the legal duty to inform the client about procedures.

> *Nursing Process:* Implementation
> *Client Needs:* Psychosocial Integrity
> *Clinical Area:* Surgical Nursing

69. (2) Two to 3 stools/day indicates that the lactulose is working to acidify the colon contents and reduce blood ammonia. If watery diarrhea occurs, there is a drug overdose.

> *Nursing Process:* Evaluation
> *Client Needs:* Physiological Integrity
> *Clinical Area:* Medical Nursing

70. (3) Mechanical ventilation may cause stress ulcers, so checking the pH to maintain it above 5 will yield information about whether or not the client requires antacids. Below 5, the pH would be too acidic and this condition could cause a stress ulcer.

> *Nursing Process:* Planning
> *Client Needs:* Physiological Integrity
> *Clinical Area:* Medical Nursing

71. (2) Normal capillary refill time is 3 seconds or less. Prolonged refill time is indicative of circulatory impairment.

> *Nursing Process:* Data Collection
> *Client Needs:* Physiological Integrity
> *Clinical Area:* Medical Nursing

72. (1) A safety measure is to have the container high enough (18 inches) to infuse, but not so high that it will infuse rapidly and cause cramps. Rapid infusion will also limit the amount of fluid the client can tolerate and retain.

Nursing Process: Implementation
Client Needs: Safe, Effective Care Environment
Clinical Area: Medical Nursing

73. (3) Elderly senile clients are often anxious, especially in an unfamiliar environment. Structure decreases anxiety. Making choices and constantly changing activities will increase anxiety. Their activity should not necessarily be limited.

Nursing Process: Planning
Client Needs: Psychosocial Integrity
Clinical Area: Psychiatric Nursing

74. (1) Denial is the first stage in the grief process. The client does not yet fully comprehend the loss that has occurred. He is protecting himself from painful feelings.

Nursing Process: Evaluation
Client Needs: Psychosocial Integrity
Clinical Area: Surgical Nursing

75. (4) The client is encouraged to express his feelings. This may lead to further discussion of the client's reactions to his own feelings when he feels threatened. Answers (2) and (3) are incorrect and focus on the intellectual aspect of this reaction. Answer (1) is incorrect because it does not encourage the client to express his feelings and explore his behavior.

Nursing Process: Implementation
Client Needs: Psychosocial Integrity
Clinical Area: Psychiatric Nursing

76. (3) High blood pressure is one of the cardinal symptoms of eclampsia, along with excessive weight gain, edema and albumin in the urine.

Nursing Process: Data Collection
Client Needs: Physiological Integrity
Clinical Area: Maternity Nursing

77. (1) Vitamin B_{12} comes from animal products. Clients with pernicious anemia have a B_{12} deficiency. Clients either need frequent B_{12} injections or they must drastically increase the foods that provide B_{12} in sufficient quantity.

Nursing Process: Evaluation
Client Needs: Health Promotion and Maintenance
Clinical Area: Medical Nursing

78. (1) Because the client cannot feel sensory stimuli, a blockage of the nerves between the central nervous system and the peripheral system is suspected.

Nursing Process: Data Collection
Client Needs: Physiological Integrity
Clinical Area: Surgical Nursing

79. (3) The nurse is sharing her observations and validating that the client looks and sounds upset, rather than asking for feedback or clarification. This technique may open communication so that the client can verbalize the fears and be more specific about the kind of help that is needed.

Nursing Process: Data Collection
Client Needs: Psychosocial Integrity
Clinical Area: Psychiatric Nursing

80. (2) The bones of a 1-year-old child are flexible and unlikely to break unless subjected to unusual stress. This could occur through child abuse; the nurse is legally responsible to report any case of suspected child abuse.

Nursing Process: Data Collection
Client Needs: Safe, Effective Care Environment
Clinical Area: Pediatric Nursing

81.   (2)   PCA works more effectively to control pain for the client with no significant difference in the amount of medication used. It is less time consuming for the nurse, but this is not the essential rationale.

> *Nursing Process:* Implementation
> *Client Needs:* Psychosocial Integrity
> *Clinical Area:* Medical Nursing

82.   (2)   Raw apples are high in potassium, while white-enriched and French bread, dry cereal, and pasta are foods low in potassium.

> *Nursing Process:* Evaluation
> *Client Needs:* Health Promotion and Maintenance
> *Clinical Area:* Medical Nursing

83.   (3)   Urecholine stimulates the parasympathetic nervous system. It increases the tone and motility of the smooth muscles of the urinary tract. It is used frequently following a TUR when the client has a lack of muscle tone and is unable to void. Bladder spasms can be relieved with Belladonna or opium suppositories.

> *Nursing Process:* Evaluation
> *Client Needs:* Safe, Effective Care Environment
> *Clinical Area:* Surgical Nursing

84.   (2)   Dose on hand is in 10 mL, so to calculate the amount to give, divide the dose desired by the dose on hand and multiply by 10 mL. Example: 0.5 gm divided by 5 gm equals 0.1, then multiplying by 10 equals 1 mL.

> *Nursing Process:* Planning
> *Client Needs:* Safe, Effective Care Environment
> *Clinical Area:* Medical Nursing

85.   (2)   The client requires treatment for shock. Vital signs are monitored after placing the client in the shock position; then the physician is called for orders.

> *Nursing Process:* Implementation
> *Client Needs:* Safe, Effective Care Environment
> *Clinical Area:* Medical Nursing

86.   (1)   When intussusception is suspected, the nurse would validate the sudden onset of symptoms because this completes the classical picture of this condition. This is one of the most frequent causes of bowel obstruction in children, especially those with celiac or cystic fibrosis disease.

> *Nursing Process:* Data Collection
> *Client Needs:* Physiological Integrity
> *Clinical Area:* Pediatric Nursing

87.   (4)   Protecting the airway from aspiration is a high priority when caring for a client receiving nasogastric tube feedings. Keeping the client in an upright position helps prevent aspiration of gastric contents. The other actions are correct but are less critical.

> *Nursing Process: Planning*
> *Client Needs:* Physiological Integrity
> *Clinical Area:* Medical Nursing

88.   (3)   Following a c-section the client will not be fed until bowel sounds are present, abdominal distention relieved, and flatus is passed. Answer (3) would be the first action followed by (2) and (4) if necessary.

> *Nursing Process:* Data Collection
> *Client Needs:* Safe, Effective Care Environment
> *Clinical Area:* Maternity Nursing

89.   (3)   Elevating the legs about 30 degrees promotes venous return and reduces leg edema. Elevation beyond 45 degrees reduces arterial flow and causes sharp flexion at the hip, thereby reducing venous return. Leaving the legs flat on the bed or dependent promotes edema formation and venous stasis. Clients with arte-

rial, rather than venous, insufficiency benefit from a dependent position.

> *Nursing Process:* Planning
> *Client Needs:* Safe, Effective Care Environment
> *Clinical Area:* Medical Nursing

90.　(4)　This response encourages the expression of feelings which may help reduce the client's anxiety. (1) does not focus on the client's feel-ings and is not a useful initial response. (2) is a closed question which discourages expression of feelings. (3) is inappropriate because it negates the client's feelings, is a stereotypical response, and expresses the nurse's opinion which is irrelevant to the situation.

> *Nursing Process:* Implementation
> *Client Needs:* Psychosocial Integrity
> *Clinical Area:* Surgical Nursing

COMPREHENSIVE TEST 4

1. A client has a disposable water-seal system with chest tubes in place. The charge nurse tells the LVN to milk the chest tubes to maintain patency. The nurse should

   1 Milk the tubes in the direction toward the client.
   2 Check that the physician has written orders to milk the chest tubes.
   3 Tell the charge nurse that this action is not appropriate for LVNs to do.
   4 Complete milking the chest tubes and chart the intervention.

2. A child is admitted with a suspected basilar skull fracture. The nurse knows that a contraindicated intervention would be to

   1 Insert a nasogastric tube.
   2 Elevate the head of the bed.
   3 Insert an endotracheal tube.
   4 Give anything by mouth until the cerebrospinal fluid leak seals.

3. A client who is a paraplegic says, "I know I shall never walk again," and begins to cry. The nurse, who feels tears in her eyes, takes his hand. The effect of this communication would be to

   1 Destroy the client's confidence in the nurse.
   2 Verify that the nurse is a very weak person.
   3 Communicate nonverbal understanding to the client.
   4 Hurt the relationship because it is an inappropriate response.

4. A client is to receive 2500 mL of IV fluid over 24 hours. The IV tubing delivers 15 gtts per 1 mL. How many drops per minute should the client receive?

   1 13 drops.
   2 26 drops.
   3 32 drops.
   4 44 drops.

5. A teenage client has been consistently late to classes, handed in assignments late and incomplete, and generally felt overwhelmed and pressured. During the client's first meeting with the nurse, she is nervous, tearful and states she is feeling inadequate. She also said she had gotten lost on the way and couldn't remember the appointment time. The nurse's best initial approach would be to

   1 Assess the client's level of anxiety.
   2 Ask the client why she is at the clinic.
   3 Reassure the client that she has come to the right place for help.
   4 Let the client set the tone for the interview.

6. A client is admitted to the CCU with a diagnosis of anterior myocardial infarction. Shortly after admission, he states, "I might as well have died because now I won't be able to do anything." The best response is

   1 "Don't worry about it, everything will be all right."
   2 "You shouldn't be thinking about that because you are doing so well now."
   3 "What do you mean about not being able to do anything?"
   4 "Take life one day at a time. It will all work out."

7. While assessing a client who has orders for a hot-water bottle, heating pad, or hot compress, the first sign of possible thermal injury is

   1 Tingling sensation in the extremities.
   2 Redness in the area.

3 Edema.

4 Pain.

8. The highest priority goal in the care of a newborn with tracheo-esophageal fistula (TEF) and esophageal atresia is to

1 Promote hydration.

2 Support maternal-infant bonding.

3 Maintain tissue integrity.

4 Maintain a patent airway.

9. A client is to receive morphine gr 1/8 IM for pain. Available is morphine 15 mg per 1 mL. The nurse would draw up

1 0.5 mL.

2 0.8 mL.

3 1.5 mL.

4 2 mL.

10. One day a client with terminal cancer says to the nurse, "Well, I've given up all hope. I know I'm going to die soon." The most therapeutic response for the nurse is to say

1 "Now, one should never give up all hope. We are finding new cures every day."

2 "We should talk about dying."

3 "You've given up all hope?"

4 "You know, your doctor will be here soon. Why don't you talk to him about your feelings."

11. The client insists on being discharged from the hospital against medical advice. From a legal standpoint, the most important nursing action is to

1 Notify the supervisor and hospital administration.

2 Determine exactly why the client wants to leave.

3 Put all appropriate forms in the client's chart before he leaves the hospital.

4 Request that the client sign the against medical advice (AMA) form.

12. A 6-month-old infant is admitted to the pediatric unit with a tentative diagnosis of dehydration. The nurse knows that early clinical signs of dehydration in infants are

1 Irritability, sunken fontanels, dry mucous membranes, and weakening peripheral pulses.

2 Rapid tachycardia, lethargy, and decreased urine output.

3 Gray skin color, poor skin turgor, bulging fontanels, and decreased urine output.

4 Lethargy, sunken fontanels, rapid respiration and pulse.

13. The client with gastric pain is advised to take antacids to relieve pain. The nurse will teach him that the antacid contraindicated for this condition is

1 Aluminum hydroxide.

2 Amphojel.

3 Maalox.

4 Soda bicarbonate.

14. The nurse is counseling a woman who has just learned she is pregnant. She says she does not want to gain too much weight because her husband likes her "thin." The most appropriate response is

1 "It's best for the baby if you don't try to stay too thin."

2 "If you are careful about the foods you eat, especially those high in calories, you will not gain too much."

3 "Let's talk about the importance of good nutrition and weight gain in pregnancy."

4 "Why don't you have your husband come to the clinic next time, and we can all talk about nutrition."

15. Which of the following statements would be accurate to make to a mother of a new baby about infant nutrition?

1 Eggs are a good source of iron and can be introduced at 6 months.

2   Solid foods can be introduced in the sixth week of life.

3   Rice cereal is the least allergenic of the cereals for infants.

4   Only one new food should be introduced per day.

16.   A client, age 60, is admitted to the hospital for a possible low intestinal obstruction. His preoperative work-up indicates vital signs of BP 100/70, P 88, R 18, and temperature of 96.4° F. Listening to bowel sounds, the nurse would expect to find

1   Absence of bowel sounds.
2   Gurgling bowel sounds.
3   Hyperactive, high-pitched sounds.
4   Tympanic, percussion sounds.

17.   A client, age 68, has an external shunt placed in preparation for hemodialysis. The nursing care plan will include

1   Observing for blood going through the shunt to identify possible clotting that may occur immediately following the dialysis run.

2   Listening for a bruit over the shunt area; if bruit is heard, the shunt may be clotted.

3   Testing the shunt to determine if it is cool to the touch, like that of the forearm, which signifies patency.

4   Observing for dark spots in the shunt that may represent clot formation.

18.   A client sustained a fracture 3 days ago. When the following blood studies are returned, they are all elevated. Which elevation would be considered a normal finding following a fracture?

1   Alkaline phosphatase.
2   Amylase.
3   Uric acid.
4   Calcium.

19.   A client with a fractured right leg has been in Buck's extension traction for a week. The nurse checking the client finds that he is now unable to dorsiflex his right foot. The nurse will notify the charge nurse because there is a possibility that the

1   Traction has been on too long.
2   Peroneal nerve function is impaired.
3   Fracture is healing with a malunion.
4   Foot is undergoing some ischemic changes.

20.   During visiting hours, a client the nurse is caring for becomes very agitated and angry with his visitor. The most effective nursing approach to this client is to

1   Restrict his visitor from coming to the hospital for a few days.

2   Approach your client in a warm, supportive manner and assist him to explore his feelings.

3   Confront your client and tell him that talking about his feelings is therapeutic.

4   Ask your client if he would like his PRN sedative in order to rest.

21.   A client was in an automobile accident and sustained a head injury. Following admission to the hospital, a diagnosis of increasing intracranial pressure was made. The nursing intervention appropriate in the care of this client is to

1   Teach controlled coughing and deep breathing.
2   Provide a quiet and brightly lit environment.
3   Elevate the head 15 to 30 degrees.
4   Encourage the intake of clear fluids.

22.   Using Leopold's maneuvers, the nurse palpates the presence of a firm round prominence over the pubic symphysis, a smooth convex structure on the client's right side, irregular structures on the left side, and a soft roundness in the fundus. The nurse would conclude that the fetal position is

1   Left occiput anterior—LOA.

2 Left occiput posterior—LOP.

3 Right occiput posterior—ROP.

4 Right occiput anterior—ROA.

23. A client who developed cerebral edema following a head injury is given mannitol (Osmitrol) intravenously. The outcome that most clearly indicates the drug has achieved its desired therapeutic effect is when the

1 Urinary output increases.

2 Client's level of awareness improves.

3 Client has no seizures.

4 Respirations drop to 12 and become regular.

24. When a client with a diagnosis of manic episode returns to the clinic to have lithium blood levels checked, her lithium level is only slightly higher than the previous week but she complains of blurred vision and ataxia. The first intervention is to

1 Withhold the next dose.

2 Instruct her to watch for signs of toxicity.

3 Notify the physician.

4 Suggest she drink more fluid.

25. A client with a healed wrist fracture has just had the cast removed. Discharge teaching by the nurse would include teaching the client to

1 Report any limb pain or swelling to the physician.

2 Perform full range of joint motion exercises to the limb.

3 Wash the limb and apply lotion liberally to the skin.

4 Discontinue elevating the limb when at rest.

26. A quadriplegic client tells the nurse that he believes he is experiencing an episode of autonomic hyperreflexia (dysreflexia). The first nursing intervention is to

1 Ask him what he thinks has precipitated this episode.

2 Assess his blood pressure and pulse.

3 Elevate his head as high as possible.

4 Assist him in emptying his bladder.

27. A 3 month old with a diagnosis of chalasia is admitted to the hospital. He has had severe weight loss because of frequent vomiting. To minimize vomiting, the nurse would place the infant

1 In a prone position after feeding.

2 On his abdomen with his head to one side.

3 On his left side with his head elevated.

4 On his right side with his head elevated.

28. Select the most effective nursing intervention for a client experiencing adult respiratory distress syndrome (ARDS).

1 Maintain low-flow oxygen via nasal cannula.

2 Encourage oral intake of at least 3000 mL fluids per day.

3 Ask open-ended questions to promote expression of anxiety.

4 Position in semi- to high-Fowler's with support to the back.

29. Which of the following behaviors would indicate improvement in coping for a client?

1 Going to the dining room to eat.

2 Initiating interaction with another client.

3 Sleeping frequently during the day.

4 Turning off the TV to listen to voices.

30. The nurse is teaching a diabetic client to monitor her blood glucose using a glucometer. The nurse will know the client is competent in performing her finger-stick to obtain blood when she

1 Uses the ball of a finger as the puncture site.

2 Uses the side of a fingertip as the puncture site.

3 Avoids using the fingers of her dominant hand as puncture sites.

4 Avoids using the thumbs as puncture sites.

31. An elderly client with the diagnosis of COPD has been admitted to the hospital. In teaching the client about his diet, which diet choice would indicate that a client with COPD understands nutritional needs?

    1 High CHO, high protein, low fat.
    2 Low CHO, high protein, high fat.
    3 High CHO, moderate protein, low fat.
    4 Moderate CHO, low protein, low fat.

32. Following delivery of a normal, healthy newborn, what is one method the nurse may implement to promote infant-mother bonding?

    1 Place the infant on the mother's abdomen.
    2 Position the baby so that mother and baby may have eye-to-eye contact.
    3 Have the lights on bright so that mother and infant can see each other.
    4 Place the infant at the mother's breast.

33. A special, controlled diet instituted relatively early after birth may prevent or limit mental retardation in children with the condition of

    1 Cretinism.
    2 Down's syndrome.
    3 Phenylketonuria (PKU).
    4 Tay-Sachs disease.

34. The nurse evaluates the results of the blood chemistry tests done on a client with acute pancreatitis. Which of the following results would the nurse expect to find?

    1 Low glucose.
    2 Low alkaline phosphatase.
    3 Elevated amylase.
    4 Elevated creatinine.

35. The nurse is completing the initial morning data collection on the client. Which physical examination technique would be used first when assessing the abdomen?

    1 Inspection.
    2 Light palpation.

3 Auscultation.
4 Percussion.

36. The LVN explains to the nursing assistant that, when obtaining an infant's respiratory rate, the NA should count respirations for 1 full minute because

    1 Young infants are abdominal breathers.
    2 Infants do not expand their lungs fully with each respiration.
    3 Activity will increase the respiratory rate.
    4 The rhythm of respiratory rate is irregular in infants.

37. A client's demand pacemaker is programmed for a ventricular rate of 72. When the nurse takes the client's apical pulse, it is 84 and regular. The nursing action is to

    1 Report this finding immediately.
    2 Obtain a cardiogram.
    3 Place the client on bedrest.
    4 Do nothing more at this time.

38. The nurse is leading a group therapy session when no one is talking and the anxiety level is increasing and the group atmosphere becoming tense. An appropriate intervention would be to

    1 Discontinue the group session.
    2 Ask the RN to join the group and help lead it.
    3 Talk about how uncomfortable it becomes when no one talks.
    4 Introduce a nonthreatening topic to talk about, such as food.

39. The nurse is caring for the mother and newborn with AIDS. An important principle of care to check that the mother understands before she leaves the hospital is to

    1 Breast-feed the infant to provide the necessary immunity.
    2 Come to the clinic for live vaccine immunization to prevent diseases.

3 Perform excellent hygiene procedures in the home.

4 Only use disinfectant soap to bathe the baby.

40. A client in labor has orders for a tocotransducer external fetal monitor to be applied. The nurse explains to the client that the purpose of this monitoring is to

1 Monitor fetal heart rate variability.
2 Quantify the strength of the contractions.
3 Record frequency and duration of contractions.
4 Obtain a tracing of the fetal cardiac cycle.

41. A client has an arteriovenous fistula as an access site for hemodialysis. Which assessment finding indicates that the fistula is patent?

1 Palpation of a pulse distal to the fistula.
2 Normal capillary refill distal to the fistula.
3 Auscultation of a bruit over the fistula.
4 Absence of edema or redness over the fistula.

42. Adequate nutrition is essential during early pregnancy for optimum fetal development. The nurse, in counseling a client, would know she understands if her daily diet includes

1 Low roughage foods.
2 One fruit or vegetable high in vitamin C.
3 A low sodium diet.
4 1500 calories.

43. A client is experiencing diarrhea as a side effect of chemotherapy. Which nursing diagnosis should receive the highest priority?

1 Fluid volume deficit.
2 Impaired skin integrity.
3 Body image disturbance.
4 Activity intolerance.

44. A 76-year-old woman who has been in good health develops urinary incontinence over a period of several days and is admitted to the hospital for a diagnostic workup. The nurse would observe the client for other indicators of

1 Renal failure.
2 Urinary tract infection.
3 Fluid volume excess.
4 Dementia.

45. At the age of 1½, a child returns to the hospital for a cleft palate repair. A very important factor in preparing the child for this experience is

1 Always allowing her a choice.
2 Never leaving her with strangers.
3 Giving her affection and a feeling of security.
4 Reminding her of her previous hospital experience.

46. The nurse teaching in a women's clinic will teach a postmenopausal woman that she is at greatest risk for the development of

1 Uterine cancer.
2 Osteoporosis.
3 Diabetes.
4 Hypertension.

47. A client tells the nurse that he is constantly under stress. The nurse could teach the client a stress reduction technique such as

1 Counting to 10 before getting angry.
2 Sitting relaxed and quiet, clearing the mind, and breathing deeply.
3 Engaging in a sport such as tennis or golf.
4 Playing a card game.

48. A pregnant client visits the clinic and asks the nurse what she can do about her legs hurting all the time. The nurse responds that the client should

1 Exercise frequently.
2 Ask the physician for medication.
3 Lie down frequently.
4 Sit or lie down with legs elevated.

49. A client had a thoracotomy and lobectomy. There are two chest tubes in place connected to a water-seal drainage system which is connected to wall suction. Which finding validates that the system is working correctly?

    1 Constant bubbling in the suction control chamber.

    2 Intermittent bubbling in the suction control chamber.

    3 Constant bubbling in the water-seal chamber.

    4 Intermittent bubbling in the drainage collection chamber.

50. A 7 year old has been diagnosed with scoliosis during a school screening. It is important for the child to have the information that

    1 It will get better with improved posture.

    2 Surgery is rarely indicated.

    3 She may wear a brace for 1 to 2 years if the scoliosis is not severe.

    4 She should avoid physical activity until after her surgery.

51. An HIV-infected client is to start on zidovudine (AZT). Which statement by the client indicates understanding of the desired therapeutic effect of this drug?

    1 "AZT will destroy the HIV virus in my body."

    2 "AZT will slow down the growth of the HIV virus."

    3 "AZT will keep me from getting infections and cancer."

    4 "AZT will prevent weight loss and fatigue."

52. Which laboratory test result would be most important to evaluate before administering a chemotherapeutic agent?

    1 Complete blood count (CBC).

    2 Liver function studies.

    3 Serum electrolytes.

    4 Prothrombin time and APTT.

53. A male client is becoming increasingly angry and verbally abusive. The *first* nursing intervention is to

    1 Send the client to his room.

    2 Place the client in restraints.

    3 Summon assistance from a male staff member.

    4 Set firm limits on the abusive behavior.

54. Teaching a new mother the principles of breast feeding, the nurse will know the mother understands how to care for her breasts when she says

    1 She will use plain soap and water to wash.

    2 After feeding, she will wash the breasts and allow them to dry.

    3 She will pull the baby off the breast frequently.

    4 She will not nurse more than every 4 hours.

55. A client is to start on finasteride (Proscar) for the treatment of benign prostatic hypertrophy (BPH). Which statement by the client indicates that he needs more teaching?

    1 "This drug will eliminate the need for prostate surgery."

    2 "I will not be surprised if I experience a decreased interest in sex."

    3 "It may take 6 or more months before this drug works."

    4 "I should be able to empty my bladder better while I'm on this drug."

56. The nurse in a well-baby clinic reminds a mother that at 4 months of age the infant should receive immunizations that include

    1 DPT, MMR and Hepatitis B.

    2 Hepatitis B only.

    3 DPT, OPV, HbCV, and HB.

    4 DPT, MMR, HbCV, and HB.

57. A newly admitted client has been diagnosed with a pulmonary embolism. The nurse would

anticipate medical orders for the immediate administration of

1 Warfarin (Coumadin).
2 Dexamethasone (Decadron).
3 Heparin.
4 Protamine sulfate.

58. A client recovering from acute pancreatitis is started on solid foods. The following dessert choices are on his menu. Which choice would indicate to the nurse that the client needs more teaching?

1 Ice cream.
2 Angel cake.
3 Canned peaches.
4 Fresh fruit cup.

59. A 7-year-old child fell off the climbing structure at school. The child is now being discharged home with a diagnosis of a mild concussion. Discharge teaching to the mother would include

1 Keeping the child on bedrest for 2 to 3 days to be sure the child doesn't hit his or her head again.
2 Giving the child nothing by mouth for at least 12 to 18 hours after the injury to be sure surgery will not be necessary.
3 Emphasizing the child's recovery may be slow and neurological sequelae are common following any head injury.
4 Closely monitoring the child (every 1 to 2 hours) for any deterioration in responsiveness.

60. Auscultation of a client's lungs reveals rales (crackles) in the left posterior base. The next intervention would be to

1 Repeat auscultation after asking the client to deep breathe and cough.
2 Instruct the client to limit fluid intake to less than 2000 mL per day.
3 Inspect the client's ankles and sacrum for the presence of edema.

4 Place the client on bedrest in a semi-Fowler's position.

61. The nurse is monitoring the following cardiac rhythms on the central cardiac monitoring console. The nurse would first assess the client whose monitor indicates

1 Atrial fibrillation.
2 Complete heart block.
3 Sinus arrhythmia.
4 Ventricular tachycardia.

62. The nurse is assigned to a client who is to have a Miller-Abbott tube inserted. Assisting the physician with this procedure, the nurse will position the client in

1 Low-Fowler's position.
2 High-Fowler's position.
3 Side-lying position.
4 Prone position.

63. The nurse finishes documenting in a chart and notices the information has been written in the wrong chart. The nurse should immediately

1 Notify the team leader so it can be initialed by an RN as a wrong entry.
2 Completely cross out the writing so it cannot be read.
3 Line out the entry with a single line, write "error" above it, and initial entry.
4 Draw a red line through the incorrect entry, write "wrong entry," and initial.

64. A pregnant multipara client presents at the clinic with painless vaginal bleeding. She is 8 months pregnant. The nursing plan would include

1 Keeping the client in bed, resting quietly.
2 Performing a vaginal examination.
3 Observing for onset of contractions.
4 Assessing for pain.

65. The nurse discovers that a surgery client drank a glass of water about 2 hours before scheduled surgery. The initial action should be to

    1 Call the operating room and cancel the surgery.
    2 Notify the charge nurse.
    3 Call the physician.
    4 Chart the occurrence on the preop check list.

66. A client is receiving the antiarrhythmic drug flecainide (Tambocor). Which nursing intervention should be implemented?

    1 Give the medication with meals.
    2 Restrict intake of high sodium foods.
    3 Monitor apical pulse rate and rhythm.
    4 Assess blood glucose by finger-stick AC and HS.

67. A physician asks the nurse to immediately administer morphine sulfate through the IV line for a client in severe pain. The correct response is

    1 "I'm sorry, I can't give the IV medication."
    2 "I will get you the medication, but I can't give the IV medication."
    3 "I'll ask the RN to give the client the medication."
    4 "I will have the RN check your order and give the IV medication STAT."

68. When assessing a child's neurological functioning, the nurse should become alarmed when

    1 A 3-month-old infant has a positive Babinski reflex.
    2 The child appears sleepy in mid-afternoon.
    3 The child is babbling incoherently.
    4 An irritable child becomes lethargic.

69. Which nursing diagnosis should receive the highest priority in a client with acute renal failure?

    1 Altered nutrition: less than body requirements related to anorexia.
    2 Risk for trauma related to decreased alertness.
    3 Activity intolerance related to fatigue and muscle cramps.
    4 Fluid volume excess related to oliguria.

70. Of the following individuals, which one cannot legally sign a consent form?

    1 A legal guardian.
    2 An emancipated minor.
    3 A pregnant teenager.
    4 The spouse.

71. The team leader LVN observes a new graduate giving a client an injection and she is not wearing gloves. When the team leader asks why she did not put on gloves, she replied, "Oh, I know this client well and he is no risk." The team leader should reply

    1 "The regulations state that all of us must wear gloves. If I see you without them, I will place you on report."
    2 "Tell me your understanding of what universal precautions for all clients means."
    3 "Well, if you are absolutely sure that you know this client—but I don't think it is safe nursing practice."
    4 "I think we should clarify this with the charge nurse to see who is right."

72. A client is hospitalized following a myocardial infarction. He is receiving Digoxin and Lasix. The teaching plan should include instruction in side effects caused by

    1 Too much sodium.
    2 Calcium loss.
    3 Potassium loss.
    4 Too much calcium.

73. A newborn is born with suspected HIV. The most important safety measure for the nurse is to

   1 Wash the infant with antibacterial soap.
   2 Wrap the infant in a clean blanket.
   3 Don gloves and gown.
   4 Teach principles of care to the mother.

74. When counseling the mother of a child with cystic fibrosis, which of the following choices would indicate to the nurse that the mother understands the most appropriate food to combine with a pancreatic enzyme?

   1 Sliced canned fruit.
   2 Cottage cheese.
   3 Applesauce.
   4 Yogurt.

75. A 3 year old in respiratory distress has orders for 90% oxygen administration. The nurse could most effectively administer this oxygen when the child is spontaneously breathing by using a(n)

   1 Oxygen tent.
   2 Face mask with rebreathing reservoir.
   3 Oxygen hood.
   4 Nasal prongs.

76. The surgeon orders a Foley catheter to be inserted. Of the following interventions, the one to carry out first would be to

   1 Clean the perineum from front to back.
   2 Check the catheter for patency.
   3 Explain the procedure to the client and tell her that she will feel slight, temporary discomfort.
   4 Arrange the sterile items on the sterile field.

77. The physician orders a nasogastric tube to be inserted. During the insertion of the NG tube, the nurse will position the client in

   1 Low-Fowler's with head tilted back.

   2 High-Fowler's with head bent forward.
   3 Right side-lying with head straight up.
   4 High-Fowler's with neck hyperextended.

78. A client needs to have a sterile urine specimen sent to the laboratory for a culture and sensitivity. After inserting the catheter, the nurse finds that urine is not flowing. The next action is to

   1 Remove the catheter, check the meatus, and reinsert the catheter.
   2 Obtain a new, larger sized catheter and insert it.
   3 Reassess if the catheter is in the vagina; if so, remove it and reinsert into meatus.
   4 Insert the catheter a little farther, wait a few seconds, and if urine does not flow, reassess placement.

79. A client comes to the emergency room and says that she has been raped. An immediate intervention is to

   1 Call the physician.
   2 Place her in a private room and remain with her.
   3 Tell her to shower and clean herself, and return to the treatment room.
   4 Call the crisis center for a rape counselor.

80. A client has just returned from a myelogram when he complains of itching and dyspnea. The nurse observes that his face is flushed. The first intervention is to

   1 Place him in low-Fowler's position.
   2 Administer oxygen at 6 l/min.
   3 Call the physician.
   4 Start an IV with normal saline.

81. Administering care to a client in hypovolemic shock, the sign that the nurse would expect to observe is

   1 Hypertension.
   2 Cyanosis.
   3 Oliguria.
   4 Tachypnea.

82. A client has been ordered to have blood work drawn for serum electrolytes. She is on bedrest and has an IV in the vein of the right forearm. The most appropriate site for blood withdrawal is the

    1 Left upper arm (brachial vein).
    2 Right forearm (radial vein).
    3 Foot (greater saphenous vein).
    4 Left forearm (median cubital vein).

83. Counseling a client on the warning signs of cancer, the nurse will describe the most dangerous lesions as

    1 Basal cell epithelioma.
    2 Squamous cell epithelioma.
    3 Malignant melanoma.
    4 Sebaceous cysts.

84. A client has burns on the front and back of both his legs and arms. The approximate percentage of his body that has been involved is

    1 27 percent.
    2 36 percent.
    3 45 percent.
    4 54 percent.

85. When performing naso-oral suctioning, the correct nursing action is to

    1 Use clean gloves and insert the catheter 6 to 8 inches into nares.
    2 Apply suction while inserting the catheter into the bronchus.
    3 Apply continuous suction as the catheter is removed during the procedure.
    4 Suction for 20 seconds and then allow a 3 minute rest period.

86. The nurse has been teaching a client to use crutches. Which statement made by the client indicates a need for more teaching?

    1 "I will not look down to watch my feet while I'm walking."
    2 "I will place my weight on the hand grips."
    3 "I will put my weak leg down first when going down stairs."
    4 "I will raise the placement of the hand grips on the crutches as I get stronger."

87. Which nursing activity is most critical in promoting the safety of a preoperative client?

    1 Assuring that a permit for surgery has been signed.
    2 Restricting the ingestion of food and fluids.
    3 Removing nail polish, lipstick, hairpins.
    4 Ensuring that the client has emptied the bladder and charting time and amount.

88. The intervention that is most helpful to minimize the incidence of orthostatic hypotension would be to

    1 Take the blood pressure before and after standing.
    2 Sit for 2 to 3 minutes before standing.
    3 Stand still for 5 to 6 minutes after rising.
    4 Walk with the client.

89. A client has recently been diagnosed with tuberculosis. The wife of the client is concerned that she will contract the disease. The nurse can teach the client's wife that the most important preventive method would be

    1 Taking the same combination of drugs her husband is taking.
    2 Not living together during the active cycle of the disease.
    3 Preventing the spread of the disease by keeping her husband in isolation when he is communicable.
    4 Taking isoniazid and vitamin B_6 for one year.

90. A client makes a suicide attempt on the evening shift. The staff intervenes in time to prevent harm. In assessing the situation, the most important rationale for the staff to discuss the incident is that

1 The staff needs to re-enact the attempt so that they understand exactly what happened.

2 The staff must file an incident report so that the hospital administration is kept informed.

3 The staff needs to discuss the client's behavior prior to the attempt to determine what cues in his behavior might have warned them that he was contemplating suicide.

4 Because the client made one suicide attempt, there is high probability he will make a second attempt in the immediate future.

COMPREHENSIVE TEST 4

Answers with Rationale

1. (2) The LVN must be sure that the physician has written orders. Stripping and milking chest tubes is allowed *only* with physician's orders because it can cause excessive negative pressure which could damage lung tissue. Chest tubes are milked away from the client toward the drainage receptacle.

    Nursing Process: Implementation
    Client Needs: Safe, Effective Care Environment
    Clinical Area: Surgical Nursing

2. (1) A nasogastric tube placement, if forced, could penetrate the fracture and intubate the brain. Elevating the head of the bed is useful in decreasing intracranial pressure. Endotracheal tubes may be necessary to maintain airway patency and breathing. The cerebrospinal fluid leak may take weeks to seal, and children are allowed oral intake as their level of consciousness and clinical status indicates.

    Nursing Process: Planning
    Client Needs: Safe, Effective Care Environment
    Clinical Area: Pediatric Nursing

3. (3) This form of nonverbal communication demonstrates the nurse sharing her humanness and understanding without becoming the focus of the interaction. It is not an inappropriate response and would strengthen, rather than hurt, the relationship.

    Nursing Process: Evaluation
    Client Needs: Psychosocial Integrity
    Clinical Area: Medical Nursing

4. (2) First, determine the number of mL to give the client each hour by dividing the total volume by the total number of hours: 2500 mL divided by 24 hours yields a desired hourly amount of 104 mL. One method for determining the minute rate uses the formula of: Volume divided by Minutes multiplied by gtts/mL equals gtts/minute. 104 divided by 60 multiplied by 15 gtts/mL equals 26 gtts/minute.

    Nursing Process: Planning
    Client Needs: Safe, Effective Care Environment
    Clinical Area: Medical Nursing

5. (1) The client is showing definite signs of anxiety and for the nurse to intervene effectively she must assess the level of anxiety. (2) is incorrect because it may add to the client's anxiety level and she needs an immediate intervention. (3) and (4) are incorrect because they do not address the client's current feelings and experiences.

    Nursing Process: Data Collection
    Client Needs: Psychosocial Integrity
    Clinical Area: Psychiatric Nursing

6. (3) By keeping the lines of communication open, the client may be able to discuss his fears and concerns. If he can verbalize these issues, he can begin to cope with his condition and continue in the rehabilitative process. The other responses close off communication.

    Nursing Process: Implementation
    Client Needs: Psychosocial Integrity
    Clinical Area: Medical Nursing

7. (2) Redness, or erythema, is the first sign of possible injury. This is an important observation to prevent a burn injury.

> *Nursing Process:* Data Collection
> *Client Needs:* Safe, Effective Care Environment
> *Clinical Area:* Medical Nursing

8. (4) The anatomical malformation in this anomaly threatens the newborn's airway. Maintaining a patent airway is the highest priority in any situation in which the airway is threatened.

> *Nursing Process:* Planning
> *Client Needs:* Safe, Effective Care Environment
> *Clinical Area:* Pediatric Nursing

9. (1) This computation can be done using the formula D (dose desired) divided by H (dose on hand) multiplied by V (volume of dose on hand) after first converting grains to milligrams. Step I: Convert grains to milligrams with 1 grain: 60 mg : : 1/8 gr : x mg. 1x = 7.5 (1/8 grain = 7.5 mg). Step II: Use formula to compute dose: 7.5 divided by 15 multiplied by 1 equals 0.5 mL.

> *Nursing Process:* Implementation
> *Client Needs:* Safe, Effective Care Environment
> *Clinical Area:* Surgical Nursing

10. (3) This reflective response will open up communication and enable the client to express whatever concerns or feelings she has without confining her to a discussion of dying (answer 2).

> *Nursing Process:* Implementation
> *Client Needs:* Psychosocial Integrity
> *Clinical Area:* Psychiatric Nursing

11. (4) All of the above actions would be appropriate to carry out. Legally, signing the against medical advice (AMA) form is most important.

> *Nursing Process:* Implementation
> *Client Needs:* Health Promotion and Maintenance
> *Clinical Area:* Medical Nursing

12. (1) Sunken fontanels, dry membranes, and weak peripheral pulses are signs of decreased extracellular fluids. Tachycardia, decreased urine output and lethargy are later findings.

> *Nursing Process:* Data Collection
> *Client Needs:* Physiological Integrity
> *Clinical Area:* Pediatric Nursing

13. (4) Soda bicarbonate is absorbed into the system and destroys acid balance; it can lead to alkalosis.

> *Nursing Process:* Implementation
> *Client Needs:* Health Promotion and Maintenance
> *Clinical Area:* Medical Nursing

14. (3) Adequate nutrition and weight gain in pregnancy are directly related to decreased mortality and morbidity in the newborn. Helping the client understand the role of nutrition and weight gain will help her then explore the best way to talk to her husband about his concerns.

> *Nursing Process:* Implementation
> *Client Needs:* Health Promotion and Maintenance
> *Clinical Area:* Maternity Nursing

15. (3) Rice cereal is the least allergic food. The latest research indicates that solid food should not be given until 6 months. This may prevent allergies later in life, and the infant's digestive system has had time to mature. Egg yolks, not whole eggs, could be introduced because the whites of the egg may cause an allergy. Each new food should be given once a week.

Nursing Process: Implementation
Client Needs: Health Promotion and Maintenance
Clinical Area: Pediatric Nursing

16. (3)   The nurse will note these sounds with an obstruction. Paralytic ileus has no bowel sounds or gurgling. Gastric distention will have tympanic sounds.

Nursing Process: Data Collection
Client Needs: Physiological Integrity
Clinical Area: Medical Nursing

17. (4)   Shunts should be inspected several times each day for presence of possible clotting. Dark spots will quickly be followed by separation of the sera and cells if clotting becomes complete. When dark spots appear, clients should be instructed to immediately seek treatment for declotting.

Nursing Process: Planning
Client Needs: Safe, Effective Care Environment
Clinical Area: Surgical Nursing

18. (1)   Bone is rich in alkaline phosphatase and blood levels normally increase following a fracture and during fracture healing. Elevation of the other blood studies should alert the nurse to the need for further assessment of the client, because of the probable presence of an illness.

Nursing Process: Evaluation
Client Needs: Physiological Integrity
Clinical Area: Surgical Nursing

19. (2)   Dorsiflexion of the foot requires an intact peroneal nerve. Compression from any part of the traction apparatus along the lateral surface of the leg just below the knee can exert pressure on the peroneal nerve and impede its function.

Nursing Process: Evaluation
Client Needs: Physiological Integrity
Clinical Area: Surgical Nursing

20. (2)   This approach would help decrease the client's anxiety and assist him in gaining insights. Answers (1) and (4) deny the problem and (3) is not as conducive to open communication.

Nursing Process: Planning
Client Needs: Psychosocial Integrity
Clinical Area: Psychiatric Nursing

21. (3)   Elevating the head promotes reduction of cerebral edema through gravity drainage. Coughing increases intracranial pressure. The environment should be nonstimulating (dim lights and quiet) to limit the risk of seizures. Fluids are restricted to avoid increasing the cerebral edema.

Nursing Process: Implementation
Client Needs: Safe, Effective Care Environment
Clinical Area: Medical Nursing

22. (4)   The head is down, the back is on the right side, legs on left, and fetus' buttocks in the fundus indicate the position of ROA.

Nursing Process: Data Collection
Client Needs: Physiological Integrity
Clinical Area: Maternity Nursing

23. (2)   Mannitol is given to reduce cerebral edema by promoting the movement of water from the tissues into the plasma followed by its excretion through the kidneys. The client's level of awareness is the most sensitive indicator of the effects of increased intracranial pressure. Improvement in the level of awareness, therefore, indicates a therapeutic response to the mannitol. The increased urinary output is simply a means through which the desired therapeutic effect is achieved. The ab-

sence of seizures does not indicate a therapeutic response to mannitol. Slowing of respirations may indicate increased cerebral edema.

> *Nursing Process:* Evaluation
> *Client Needs:* Physiological Integrity
> *Clinical Area:* Medical Nursing

24. (1) These are symptoms of toxicity and the nurse must withhold the next dose. The nurse would then notify the physician. The client needs to maintain a normal fluid level to prevent toxicity, but this may not be the cause of her symptoms.

> *Nursing Process:* Implementation
> *Client Needs:* Safe, Effective Care Environment
> *Clinical Area:* Psychiatric Nursing

25. (3) Dry skin, oil, and other debris collect under a cast and can be removed by washing the limb and keeping it lubricated. Some pain and swelling are normal after a limb is freed from the confines of a cast. The client should gently exercise the limb to the point of pain only, rather than to the point of full ROM. The limb should continue to be elevated when at rest to limit swelling.

> *Nursing Process:* Implementation
> *Client Needs:* Health Promotion and Maintenance
> *Clinical Area:* Surgical Nursing

26. (3) Blood pressure can become dangerously elevated during an episode of dysreflexia and can cause cerebral and retinal hemorrhages. Elevating the head will help prevent these complications and should be the nurse's first action. Identifying the precipitant is useful in terminating the episode by removing the noxious stimulus which provoked the exaggerated autonomic response. A full bladder may precipitate dysreflexia and emptying the bladder would be appropriate if it was the precipitant.

The blood pressure and pulse should be monitored throughout the episode of dysreflexia.

> *Nursing Process:* Implementation
> *Client Needs:* Safe, Effective Care Environment
> *Clinical Area:* Medical Nursing

27. (4) The greater curvature of the stomach is toward the left side so the right side position affords less pressure. Elevation of the head would lessen the tendency to vomit.

> *Nursing Process:* Implementation
> *Client Needs:* Safe, Effective Care Environment
> *Clinical Area:* Pediatric Nursing

28. (4) ARDS produces severe dyspnea and life-threatening abnormalities of blood gases; therefore, maintaining an upright position will promote gas exchange and help relieve dyspnea. The client with ARDS requires high concentrations of oxygen, usually by mask or ventilator. Diuretics and fluid restrictions are used to combat the pulmonary edema which is part of ARDS. Closed questions are used because of the client's dyspnea; the expected anxiety needs to be addressed through interventions other than verbalization.

> *Nursing Process:* Implementation
> *Client Needs:* Safe, Effective Care Environment
> *Clinical Area:* Medical Nursing

29. (2) If a client can initiate interaction with another client, it indicates he is not totally absorbed in himself, too depressed to initiate, or too absorbed in delusions or hallucinations to interact. All of the other choices do not indicate improvement in coping.

> *Nursing Process:* Evaluation
> *Client Need:* Psychosocial Integrity
> *Clinical Area:* Psychiatric Nursing

30. (2) The sides of fingertips have fewer nerve endings than do the balls of the finger, so less discomfort will result from selecting the sides as puncture sites. Both hands, including the thumbs, can be used as puncture sites.

> *Nursing Process:* Evaluation
> *Client Needs:* Health Promotion and Maintenance
> *Clinical Area:* Medical Nursing

31. (2) Carbohydrate metabolism produces carbon dioxide which increases the blood levels of carbon dioxide. High protein prevents muscle wasting and helps preserve the strength of muscles, including the muscles of respiration. Calorie and energy needs are met by increasing the fat intake.

> *Nursing Process:* Evaluation
> *Client Needs:* Health Promotion and Maintenance
> *Clinical Area:* Medical Nursing

32. (2) The most effective method of initial bonding is eye-to-eye contact. The lights should be dimmed so that the infant can open eyes fully. Placing the infant at the mother's breast will contribute to bonding (and to uterine contractions), but is not the most important method.

> *Nursing Process:* Implementation
> *Client Needs:* Psychosocial Integrity
> *Clinical Area:* Maternity Nursing

33. (3) A strictly controlled diet, eliminating protein because the infant cannot metabolize the amino acid, phenylalanine, will prevent or limit mental retardation. A special formula is used for the infant and a special diet must be followed until adulthood.

> *Nursing Process:* Planning
> *Client Needs:* Health Promotion and Maintenance
> *Clinical Area:* Pediatric Nursing

34. (3) Amylase is produced by the pancreas. An inflamed pancreas is unable to adequately secrete the amylase into the intestinal tract producing elevated levels of amylase in the blood. Glucose and alkaline phosphatase are also likely to be elevated in acute pancreatitis. Creatinine is unaffected by acute pancreatitis.

> *Nursing Process:* Evaluation
> *Client Needs:* Physiological Integrity
> *Clinical Area:* Medical Nursing

35. (1) Visual inspection is the first step in assessing the abdomen. Auscultation is next because palpation or percussion can alter bowel motility, thereby producing inaccurate findings.

> *Nursing Process:* Data Collection
> *Client Needs:* Safe, Effective Care Environment
> *Clinical Area:* Medical Nursing

36. (4) Infants breathe in an irregular pattern with varying depth and rate so that a one minute count is appropriate. (1), (2) and (3) are true statements, but not the correct answer.

> *Nursing Process:* Data Collection
> *Client Needs:* Health Promotion and Maintenance
> *Clinical Area:* Pediatric Nursing

37. (4) A demand pacemaker stimulates cardiac contraction when the heart rate falls below the preset rate. A regular rate that is above the demand rate and below 100 indicates that the client's heart is beating independently at a normal sinus rate; therefore, no action is called for at this time.

> *Nursing Process:* Implementation
> *Client Needs:* Safe, Effective Care Environment
> *Clinical Area:* Medical Nursing

38. (3) It is appropriate to comment on what is happening now—this will also reduce the anxiety. Options (1) and (2) are inappropriate because it seems as if the nurse is unable to handle the group. Answer (4) is superficial and is not dealing with the issue.

> *Nursing Process:* Implementation
> *Client Needs:* Psychosocial Integrity
> *Clinical Area:* Psychiatric Nursing

39. (3) The most important guideline is for the mother to use excellent hygiene procedures, including handwashing, to prevent transmitting the disease and infection. The mother would probably be counseled not to breastfeed and the baby would not be given live vaccines if infected with AIDS. It is not necessary to use disinfectant soap.

> *Nursing Process:* Evaluation
> *Client Needs:* Health Promotion and Maintenance
> *Clinical Area:* Maternity Nursing

40. (3) The purpose of this tocotransducer monitor is to provide tracings of uterine activity. This type of monitor does not record fetal heart rate variability or quantify the contraction strength. Only an internal fetal electrode will provide a tracing of the fetal cardiac cycle and beat-to-beat variability.

> *Nursing Process:* Implementation
> *Client Needs:* Health Promotion and Maintenance
> *Clinical Area:* Maternity Nursing

41. (3) The flow of blood through a patent arteriovenous fistula produces turbulence manifested by a bruit audible when the fistula is auscultated.

> *Nursing Process:* Data Collection
> *Client Needs:* Safe, Effective Care Environment
> *Clinical Area:* Medical Nursing

42. (2) The diet must include at least one fruit or vegetable high in vitamin C, and should include a total of four fruits and vegetables. Pregnancy requires the addition of 300 calories a day over regular caloric intake, and 1500 calories a day would be inadequate. The recommended calories for someone age 28 are 2300 a day. Research indicates that sodium is essential during pregnancy.

> *Nursing Process:* Evaluation
> *Client Needs:* Health Promotion and Maintenance
> *Clinical Area:* Maternity Nursing

43. (1) Although all of these nursing diagnoses could apply to a client with diarrhea, fluid volume deficit is the priority diagnosis because it is potentially life-threatening.

> *Nursing Process:* Planning
> *Client Needs:* Physiological Integrity
> *Clinical Area:* Medical Nursing

44. (2) Urinary tract infections in the elderly often present as urinary incontinence that develops suddenly. Renal failure and fluid volume excess typically are characterized by oliguria. Dementia develops slowly and is manifested by disordered thinking and behavior.

> *Nursing Process:* Data Collection
> *Client Needs:* Physiological Integrity
> *Clinical Area:* Medical Nursing

45. (3) A child needs extra assurance at this age. Children suffer separation anxiety and need to feel that someone is close to protect them.

> *Nursing Process:* Planning
> *Client Needs:* Health Promotion and Maintenance
> *Clinical Area:* Pediatric Nursing

46. (2) The decrease in estrogen which occurs after menopause creates a high risk for the development of osteoporosis. The other health

problems may occur, but research does not indicate they are related to hormone levels.

> *Nursing Process:* Implementation
> *Client Needs:* Health Promotion and Maintenance
> *Clinical Area:* Maternity Nursing

47. (2) Meditation or just sitting quietly, breathing deeply, and keeping the mind clear is a very effective stress reduction technique. The other choices are not considered stress reducers—sports or games that are competitive may create even more stress.

> *Nursing Process:* Planning
> *Client Needs:* Health Promotion and Maintenance
> *Clinical Area:* Psychiatric Nursing

48. (4) The best relief measure for varicosities or edema in the legs (which could cause pain) is to elevate them while sitting or lying down. Medication would not be appropriate.

> *Nursing Process:* Implementation
> *Client Needs:* Health Promotion and Maintenance
> *Clinical Area:* Maternity Nursing

49. (1) When a water-seal drainage system is connected to a suction source, there should be continuous bubbling in the suction control chamber. All of the other assessment findings indicate some form of malfunction in the system.

> *Nursing Process:* Evaluation
> *Client Needs:* Safe, Effective Care Environment
> *Clinical Area:* Surgical Nursing

50. (3) Bracing can effectively stop the progression of mild scoliosis, while posture will not change structural scoliosis. Surgery is indicated for severe scoliosis and when the curve increases as the child grows. Physical activity does not need to be restricted before surgery.

> *Nursing Process:* Implementation
> *Client Needs:* Health Promotion and Maintenance
> *Clinical Area:* Pediatric Nursing

51. (2) AZT inhibits the replication of the HIV virus, thereby slowing the rate of growth of the virus. It does not completely destroy the virus nor does it universally prevent infections, cancer or other manifestations of HIV/AIDS.

> *Nursing Process:* Evaluation
> *Client Needs:* Physiological Integrity
> *Clinical Area:* Medical Nursing

52. (1) Chemotherapy commonly results in bone marrow depression. The CBC is evaluated to determine the adequacy of bone marrow function. Low WBC or platelet counts can be indicators of life-threatening toxicity.

> *Nursing Process:* Planning
> *Client Needs:* Safe, Effective Care Environment
> *Clinical Area:* Medical Nursing

53. (4) The first intervention would be to calmly set limits to defuse the situation. The nurse would not place the client in restraints until he is totally out of control; nor would the nurse summon a male staff member initially —a sudden involvement of others could escalate the situation. After the initial intervention, the client could be sent to his room.

> *Nursing Process:* Implementation
> *Client Needs:* Safe, Effective Care Environment
> *Clinical Area:* Psychiatric Nursing

54. (2) The breasts need to be dried after feeding. No soap should be used because it removes natural oils. The baby should not be

pulled off the breast because it will make the breast sore. The baby should not be nursed more than every 2 hours.

Nursing Process: Evaluation
Client Needs: Health Promotion and Maintenance
Clinical Area: Maternity Nursing

55. (1) Because this statement is incorrect, the client will need more teaching. Finasteride is an androgen inhibitor which may promote a reduction of prostatic hypertrophy, thereby improving bladder emptying. It may take 6 to 12 months to become effective and it does not work for all clients. Some clients, therefore, will need surgery to relieve the obstructive symptoms of BPH. One of the side effects of the drug is decreased libido.

Nursing Process: Evaluation
Client Needs: Health Promotion and Maintenance
Clinical Area: Medical Nursing

56. (3) At 4 months, most children receive DPT, (diphtheria, pertussis and tetanus toxoid); trivalent oral polio vaccine; hemophilus influenzae type b; and hepatitis B. MMR (measles, mumps and rubella) is given at 15 months and 11 to 12 years. This is recommended by the Schedule Committee on Infectious Disease from the American Academy of Pediatrics.

Nursing Process: Planning
Client Needs: Health Promotion and Maintenance
Clinical Area: Pediatric Nursing

57. (3) Heparin acts rapidly to prevent extension of emboli and the formation of thrombi. Warfarin is a slow-acting anticoagulant. Protamine sulfate inactivates heparin. Dexamethasone, a corticosteroid, is not indicated for the immediate treatment of pulmonary embolism.

Nursing Process: Planning
Client Needs: Physiological Integrity
Clinical Area: Medical Nursing

58. (1) Infection or inflammation of the pancreas or biliary tract impairs the ability to digest fats. High fat foods such as ice cream should be avoided. The other selections are low in fat.

Nursing Process: Evaluation
Client Needs: Health Promotion and Maintenance
Clinical Area: Medical Nursing

59. (4) Recovery is usually rapid and complete, but frequent, careful monitoring initially will detect signs of a more serious injury. Activity and fluids are advised as tolerated. The child does not necessarily have to be on bedrest.

Nursing Process: Planning
Client Needs: Health Promotion and Maintenance
Clinical Area: Pediatric Nursing

60. (1) Although rales (crackles) often indicate fluid in the alveoli, they may also be related to hypoventilation and will clear after a deep breath or a cough. It is, therefore, premature to impose fluid or activity restrictions. Inspection for edema would be appropriate after reauscultation.

Nursing Process: Implementation
Client Needs: Safe, Effective Care Environment
Clinical Area: Medical Nursing

61. (4) Ventricular tachycardia is a life threatening arrhythmia because it severely limits cardiac output and can degenerate quickly into ventricular fibrillation. Although atrial fibrillation and complete heart block can limit cardiac output, they are not as immediately life

threatening as is ventricular tachycardia. Sinus arrhythmia is not life threatening.

> *Nursing Process:* Data Collection
> *Client Needs:* Safe, Effective Care Environment
> *Clinical Area:* Medical Nursing

62. (2) High-Fowler's with neck flexed is the position necessary for tube insertion, as it is inserted through the nose into the intestine.

> *Nursing Process:* Implementation
> *Client Needs:* Safe, Effective Care Environment
> *Clinical Area:* Medical Nursing

63. (3) A single line through the entry with the word "error" above and the nurse's initials following is the correct method to indicate an incorrect chart entry has occurred.

> *Nursing Process:* Implementation
> *Client Needs:* Safe, Effective Care Environment
> *Clinical Area:* Medical Nursing

64. (1) The most important goal is to maintain the client in bed, resting quietly because the symptom, painless bleeding, may indicate placenta previa. With this symptom, a vaginal examination would not be done.

> *Nursing Process:* Planning
> *Client Needs:* Physiological Integrity
> *Clinical Area:* Maternity Nursing

65. (2) Notify the charge nurse so he/she can notify the physician to obtain further orders.

> *Nursing Process:* Implementation
> *Client Needs:* Safe, Effective Care Environment
> *Clinical Area:* Surgical Nursing

66. (3) Flecainide is an antiarrhythmic used for the treatment of certain life-threatening ar-

rhythmias. The apical pulse is monitored to evaluate the therapeutic response to the drug and to detect any new arrhythmias which may represent a side or toxic effect of this potent drug.

> *Nursing Process:* Evaluation
> *Client Needs:* Safe, Effective Care Environment
> *Clinical Area:* Medical Nursing

67. (4) The best response is (4). An LVN may not give IV medications, nor give an RN a verbal order from a physician.

> *Nursing Process:* Implementation
> *Client Needs:* Safe, Effective Care Environment
> *Clinical Area:* Medical Nursing

68. (4) A change from irritability to lethargy signals serious central nervous system deterioration and demands *immediate* action. Babinski signs often persist until the child begins to walk. The time of day should be considered when evaluating neurological function because children can appear lethargic at usual sleep times. The age of the child should be considered when assessing language.

> *Nursing Process:* Data Collection
> *Client Needs:* Physiological Integrity
> *Clinical Area:* Pediatric Nursing

69. (4) The oliguria associated with acute renal failure results in fluid volume excess. The increase in fluid volume may produce life-threatening effects such as heart failure, hypertension, and cerebral edema. The other nursing diagnoses would have lower priority.

> *Nursing Process:* Planning
> *Client Needs:* Physiological Integrity
> *Clinical Area:* Medical Nursing

70. (4) In most situations, a spouse cannot sign a consent to treatment. If a person is not determined to be legally competent to sign the doc-

ument, the spouse may be assigned as the legal guardian or conservator.

> *Nursing Process:* Planning
> *Client Needs:* Safe, Effective Care Environment
> *Clinical Area:* Surgical Nursing

71. (2)   The best way to determine what the new graduate knows and/or understands is to ask this basic question. Once the team leader has baseline data, then teaching about the importance of always using universal precautions can be done. Universal precautions are to be used for *all* clients when there is a danger of coming into contact with body fluids.

> *Nursing Process:* Implementation
> *Client Needs:* Health Promotion and Maintenance
> *Clinical Area:* Medical Nursing

72. (3)   Lasix is a loop diuretic which inhibits the reabsorption of sodium and chloride in the ascending loop of Henle. Potassium loss is a direct result of a large volume of urine output. The client should be taught the symptoms of hypokalemia. The client will not be hyper- or hypocalcemic or necessarily have a high sodium level because of the Lasix.

> *Nursing Process:* Planning
> *Client Needs:* Health Promotion and Maintenance
> *Clinical Area:* Medical Nursing

73. (3)   Universal precautions are the most important safety measures, so donning gloves and gown with all newborns is necessary. The infant would be washed with Neutrogena soap. The other actions would be performed, but are not the most important.

> *Nursing Process:* Planning
> *Client Needs:* Safe, Effective Care Environment
> *Clinical Area:* Maternity Nursing

74. (3)   Enzymes cannot be mixed with proteins. Mixing the enzyme in a small amount of applesauce allows the child to swallow it easily. Most children like applesauce so it is not as difficult to get them to swallow it.

> *Nursing Process:* Evaluation
> *Clinical Area:* Health Promotion and Maintenance
> *Client Needs:* Medical Nursing

75. (2)   Up to 100% oxygen flow is possible with the seal of the mask and reservoir. Other methods listed deliver only a maximum of 40% oxygen.

> *Nursing Process:* Planning
> *Client Needs:* Safe, Effective Care Environment
> *Clinical Area:* Pediatric Nursing

76. (3)   Giving the client an adequate explanation for the procedure will result in less anxiety and more cooperation.

> *Nursing Process:* Implementation
> *Client Needs:* Psychosocial Integrity
> *Clinical Area:* Surgical Nursing

77. (2)   The preferred position is Fowler's with the head flexed forward to assist the tube to move into the esophagus. The nurse would never ask the client to hyperextend the neck, as this might open the airway and cause the tube to enter the trachea.

> *Nursing Process:* Implementation
> *Client Needs:* Safe, Effective Care Environment
> *Clinical Area:* Medical Nursing

78. (4)   Check if catheter is inserted far enough into urethra or if it is in vagina. If in vagina, leave in place as a landmark, obtain new sterile set-up, and insert new catheter.

Nursing Process: Implementation
Client Needs: Safe, Effective Care
Environment
Clinical Area: Medical Nursing

79. (2) The immediate intervention is to provide privacy and remain with the victim for support. The nurse would not allow the client to wash because the goal is to preserve existing evidence. The next step is to prepare the client for a complete physical exam and call the physician. Rape counseling would come later.

   Nursing Process: Implementation
   Client Needs: Psychosocial Integrity
   Clinical Area: Psychiatric Nursing

80. (1) Low-Fowler's position promotes optimal perfusion and adequate ventilatory exchange. Oxygen administration is the second nursing intervention.

   Nursing Process: Implementation
   Client Needs: Safe, Effective Care
   Environment
   Clinical Area: Medical Nursing

81. (3) In shock, there is decreased blood volume through the kidneys. This is evidenced by a decrease in the amount of urine excreted. The body has numerous compensatory mechanisms that assist in keeping the blood pressure normal for a short time.

   Nursing Process: Data Collection
   Client Needs: Physiological Integrity
   Clinical Area: Medical Nursing

82. (4) Blood should be drawn from the most peripheral vein to preserve the integrity of the vein for future lab work. With an IV in the right forearm, this site would be unacceptable for blood withdrawal.

Nursing Process: Data Collection
Client Needs: Safe, Effective Care
Environment
Clinical Area: Medical Nursing

83. (3) Melanoma is the most dangerous. A sebaceous cyst is a benign (nonmalignant) growth. Basal cell epithelioma and squamous cell epithelioma are both superficial, easily excised, slow-growing tumors.

   Nursing Process: Implementation
   Client Needs: Physiological Integrity
   Clinical Area: Medical Nursing

84. (4) The client's burns cover approximately 54 percent of his body surface. Each arm is 9 percent (18 percent) and each leg is 18 percent (36 percent).

   Nursing Process: Data Collection
   Client Needs: Physiological Integrity
   Clinical Area: Medical Nursing

85. (1) Clean, rather than sterile, gloves can be used for naso-oral suctioning and the nurse would insert the catheter through the nares without applying suction. Suctioning is limited to 10 seconds to prevent excessive removal of oxygen. Suction on the catheter is released intermittently during the procedure and when being withdrawn.

   Nursing Process: Implementation
   Client Need: Safe, Effective Care
   Environment
   Clinical Area: Surgical Nursing

86. (4) The hand grips should be placed so that the elbows are flexed at 20 to 30 degrees when standing with the crutches. This placement should not be changed as long as the client continues to need crutches. The other statements indicate effective learning.

Nursing Process: Evaluation
Client Needs: Health Promotion and Maintenance
Clinical Area: Surgical Nursing

87. (2) Restricting food and fluids helps protect the client's airway by preventing aspiration of vomitus while under anesthesia. The other actions are correct but are less critical.

> *Nursing Process:* Planning
> *Client Needs:* Safe, Effective Care Environment
> *Clinical Area:* Surgical Nursing

88. (2) A drop in blood pressure commonly occurs when changing from a recumbent to upright position, causing blood to pool in the lower body. Sitting up before standing lets the body adjust the flow of blood and redirects some of the blood back to the upper body and brain. Walking with the client does not prevent development of this problem.

> *Nursing Process:* Planning
> *Client Needs:* Physiological Integrity
> *Clinical Area:* Medical Nursing

89. (4) Those people infected with the tubercle bascillus without the disease and those at high risk for developing the disease should receive a drug regimen of isoniazid and vitamin B_6 as prophylaxis. Measures to prevent the spread of the disease should also be implemented; but, depending on the relationship, not living with her husband or keeping him in isolation are not the usual methods.

> *Nursing Process:* Implementation
> *Client Needs:* Health Promotion and Maintenance
> *Clinical Area:* Medical Nursing

90. (3) Even though all of the reasons are important and should not be ignored, the most important task for the staff is to assess the client's behavior and to identify cues that might indicate an impending suicide attempt.

> *Nursing Process:* Data Collection
> *Client Needs:* Psychosocial Integrity
> *Clinical Area:* Psychiatric Nursing

VII

SELF-ASSESSMENT AND EVALUATION GRIDS

COMPREHENSIVE TESTS 3 & 4

Grid I Comprehensive Texts 3 & 4		Clinical Area					
		Medical Nursing	Surgical Nursing	Maternity Nursing	Pediatric Nursing	Psychiatric Nursing	Total Answers Wrong
Nursing Process	Data Collection						
	Planning						
	Implementation						
	Evaluation						
	Total Answers Wrong						

Grid II Comprehensive Texts 3 & 4		Clinical Area					
		Medical Nursing	Surgical Nursing	Maternity Nursing	Pediatric Nursing	Psychiatric Nursing	Total Answers Wrong
Client Needs	**Safe, Effective Care Environment**						
	Physiological Integrity						
	Psychosocial Integrity						
	Health Promotion and Maintenance						
	Total Answers Wrong						

Information About Your Computer Disk

The 3.5-inch IBM-compatible computer disk attached to the inside back cover of your book offers you the opportunity to rehearse taking the NCLEX. You use the same computer keys to operate the program as when actually taking the NCLEX. Reading questions on the screen and using the keyboard for answer selection will increase your comfort level with computer testing and boost your confidence as well. Additional helpful information about Computerized Adaptive Testing and NCLEX procedures is contained in the Introduction to this book.

The 100 simulated NCLEX-PN CAT questions on the disk are based on the current NCLEX Test Plan and the most recent Job Analysis of new graduate nurses. This program is very easy to use. The disk runs on the DOS operating system of IBM and IBM-compatible computers. Your computer needs only a minimum of 512K memory and a 3.5-inch floppy drive.

Starting Your Program

1. Insert the disk into the floppy drive and type **A:** or **B:** (depending on the configuration of your equipment) and press **Enter**

2. Type **BEGIN** and press **Enter**

   The introductory screens familiarize you with how the program operates and lists the options on the Main Menu. You can interrupt the test and return to the next unanswered question at any time.

Feedback

In the **Practice Mode**, you will receive feedback—correct or incorrect plus the rationale—immediately after answering each question. In the **Test Mode**, you will answer all 100 questions on the disk before obtaining your results.

Upon completing the test in either mode, you can obtain a Performance Summary that includes your overall score on the test and a breakdown of your results in terms of Nursing Process, Client Needs, and Clinical Area. This information, which can be displayed on the screen or printed out, provides you with clues concerning where you should focus additional study and review. You also have the option of reviewing the questions you answered incorrectly along with their rationales. When finished, you can clear the disk and begin again. There are no limitations on the number of times that you can use this disk.

Problem Solving

If you experience a problem operating the disk, check the following:

1. Make sure you are running the program on DOS, not Windows. The program may not run through Windows. If your computer is set up to process your applications through Windows, return to the basic DOS prompt before starting the program.

2. If you have copied the files from the disk to your hard drive, try running the program directly from the disk.

3. Make sure that the write protect window (small tab on the upper corner of the disk) is closed.

4. If the Performance Summary does not appear upon command, you did not answer all the questions. You must complete the test before obtaining your Performance Summary.

If you continue to experience problems operating the program, contact Viacom/Simon & Schuster c/o Starpack, 237 22nd Street, Greeley, CO 80631 (800) 991-0077.